María Elisa Sarmiento de Cannata
Nancy Roxana Vera
Silvia Nelina González

PHARMACOVIGILANCE

María Elisa Sarmiento de Cannata
Nancy Roxana Vera
Silvia Nelina González

PHARMACOVIGILANCE

Ecological medicine in the drug chain

ScienciaScripts

Imprint
Any brand names and product names mentioned in this book are subject to trademark, brand or patent protection and are trademarks or registered trademarks of their respective holders. The use of brand names, product names, common names, trade names, product descriptions etc. even without a particular marking in this work is in no way to be construed to mean that such names may be regarded as unrestricted in respect of trademark and brand protection legislation and could thus be used by anyone.

Cover image: www.ingimage.com

This book is a translation from the original published under ISBN 978-613-9-40470-4.

Publisher:
Sciencia Scripts
is a trademark of
Dodo Books Indian Ocean Ltd. and OmniScriptum S.R.L publishing group

120 High Road, East Finchley, London, N2 9ED, United Kingdom
Str. Armeneasca 28/1, office 1, Chisinau MD-2012, Republic of Moldova, Europe
Printed at: see last page
ISBN: 978-620-8-29368-0

PHARMACOVIGILANCE

Ecological medicine in the drug chain

María Elisa Sarmiento de Cannata

Nancy R. Vera

Silvia N. González

Acknowledgment

I thank God for giving me the opportunity to write this thesis, as a contribution to the university educational institution where I was a student and teacher; to my husband, my partner in life and projects; to Pipe for his illustration that represents my work; and to the professionals who accompanied me in this scientific adventure.

Index

Summary

The medicine used by an urban population for different purposes, including therapeutic ones, becomes a pollutant when it enters a natural ecosystem, alters its balance, affects its health and turns an environment that provides natural resources (water and food of plant and animal origin) into a danger to human health. This work begins the study of pharmacovigilance in the Salí Dulce watershed, with the detection of modifications in the state of health of this eco-system that endanger biodiversity, sustainability and human health; to later search for the presence of non-biodegradable organic molecules as potential active pharmaceutical ingredients (API).

The standard techniques used qualitatively and quantitatively, as well as the complementary techniques of infrared spectroscopy with Fourier transform and atomic spectrometry with high detection sensitivity, were useful for the construction of an analytical and then holistic knowledge of the delimited ecosystem. Detecting an altered self-purification in the water ecosystem, plus the presence of organic molecules moving in the water of the Basin, indicate the loss of the system's capacity to free itself from them; this justifies the need to continue the environmental study, with the purpose of identifying biologically active molecules and establishing their concentration.

Our findings show the need for pharmacovigilance activities in the Basin under study, associated with educational strategies related to the use of medicines at each stage of their life cycle, which largely takes place in the social structure known as the Medicine Chain. It is necessary to involve the actors of the Drug Chain, for an efficient use in each link of the chain, which requires responsibility and prudence. Pharmacovigilance becomes a useful tool for Ecological Medicine, which, by caring for the health of the environment, cares for the health of the population, chronically and inadvertently exposed to biologically active molecules.

Keywords: Salí Dulce watershed; Ecological medicine; Pharmacologically active ingredient.

Chapter 1

Freshwater chemical contaminants

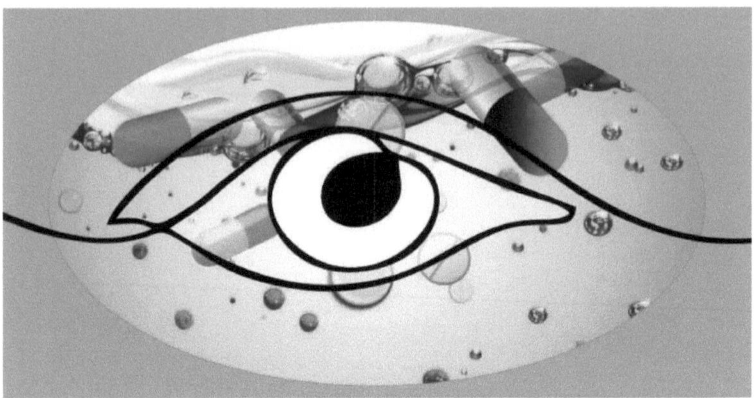

1.1 Definition of Contamination
1.2 Types of Water Pollution
1.3 Behavior of organic substances in the environment
1.4 Behavior of non-biodegradable organic substances: ***Emerging*** *Contaminants*
1.5 Active Pharmaceutical Ingredients in the aquatic environment.
1.6 Pharmacokinesis of chemical contaminants
1.7 Pharmacodynamics of chemical contaminants
1.8 Bibliography

1.1 Pollution - Definition

The action and effect of contaminating and becoming contaminated, i.e. to harmfully alter the purity or normal conditions of a thing or a medium by chemical or physical agents A pollutant is a substance that appears in the environment as a result of human activities and has a harmful effect on the environment.

Environmental pollution [Cattogio 1993] is a state of disturbance that limits the sustainable development of a community. It can be produced by physical, chemical or biological agents (pollutants) that interact with different levels of organization of the biota, in a way that is harmful to human, animal or plant life.

Chemical pollution may be due to the appearance of a new substance in a natural system (atmosphere, water, soil) or to an increase in the concentration of a substance in the system, exceeding typical and natural variations, which causes damage to human, animal or plant life and negatively alters the natural balance.

The toxicity of contaminants will depend on their chemical characteristics, concentration, and persistence in the environment. Some disappear from the environment very quickly, it is said that they have a short half-life, i.e. 50% of the toxic form of the pollutant disappears, others persist in the environment for decades.

Chemical pollution has a negative impact on health, on life and on the performance of productive activities such as agriculture and livestock farming, where water is an essential element.

Water is a scarce natural resource, indispensable for human life and environmental sustainability, which, as a result of rapid human and economic development and the inappropriate use of water as a means of disposal, has suffered an alarming deterioration.

Pollution, which changes water quality and disturbs or destroys natural resources, can cause health risks and affect aquatic communities.

1.2 Types of Water Pollution

Toxic inorganic substances: originating from industry and mining, for example heavy metals, dispersants, etc. These are acids, salts or toxic metals, such as mercury or lead, whose presence in water can cause serious damage to aquatic ecosystems, reducing biodiversity. They come from domestic, agricultural and industrial discharges, which may contain various chemical compounds.

Contamination with heavy metals: this is one of the most dangerous forms of environmental contamination, firstly because it does not present any possible chemical or biological degradation, and also because it can be bioaccumulated in different ways and remain in organisms for long periods of time.

The usual sources of wastewater contain large amounts of metals such as chromium, cadmium, copper, mercury, lead and zinc, which have the following effects on the environment: mortality of plankton, mollusks and fish, and also accumulate in the sediment.

Another series of metals such as iron, calcium, magnesium or manganese are also present in industrial wastewater, their effects, less dangerous than the previous ones, are responsible for the change in water characteristics: color, hardness, salinity and incrustations.

Toxic organic substances: The behavior of organic compounds depends on their molecular structure, size, the presence of functional groups that are important determinants of toxicity.

It is necessary to know the structure of organic compounds in order to predict their fate in living organisms and in the environment.

Contaminating organic molecules are classified according to their origin:

-Natural organic molecules are those synthesized by living organisms and those derived from petroleum such as hydrocarbons. Hydrocarbons are compounds containing only carbon and hydrogen. They are divided into two classes: aliphatic and aromatic hydrocarbons. The latter are much more reactive than aliphatic hydrocarbons.
-Man-made organic molecules: these are substances that do not exist in nature and have been manufactured or synthesized by man, e.g. plastics, pharmaceuticals, deodorants, perfumes, detergents, soaps, synthetic textile fibers, polymers in general, or organic dyes [Halden 2015].

1.3 Behavior of organic substances in the environment

Biodegradable organic substances are provided by primary producers (via photosynthesis) and by the vital processes of living organisms, including man. Non-biodegradable organic substances result from anthropogenic processes (exploitation of fossil fuels, industrial production, agriculture, animal husbandry, etc.) and include organochlorine pesticides and polychlorinated biphenyls.

1.4 Behavior of non-biodegradable organic substances: Emerging Contaminants

Of anthropogenic origin. E.g. biocides [Dhillon et al., 2015], dyes (anilines), hydrocarbons, etc. Synthetic organic compounds, which are difficult to biodegrade, include halogenated pesticides, organochlorines, biphenylpolychlorines, polycyclic aromatic hydrocarbons.

Persistent Organic Pollutants (POPs)

They are characterized by the following environmental performance:

-Low solubility in water and high in lipids so they can pass through biological membranes and accumulate in fat deposits, mainly in fish and mammals: bioaccumulation.

-Persistent in the environment. Very high residence time in the environment: resistant to photolytic, biological and chemical degradation.

-Propagation to other geographical locations

Bioaccumulation alters the food chain, causing predators to consume contaminated prey; thus, humans can be exposed to chemical contaminants by eating contaminated fish; if the contaminant persists in the aquatic environment, exposure occurs through drinking water or recreational activities.

In addition, they can generate biomagnification by accumulating at higher levels of the food chain.

There are organic pollutants that are persistent in the environment, due to their continuous entry, as is the case of emerging pollutants of urban origin such as detergents that produce foams and add phosphate to the water (eutrophication), thus greatly diminishing the self-purifying power of rivers by hindering bacterial activity. They also interfere in the flocculation and sedimentation processes in the treatment plants.

Emerging Contaminants in the aquatic environment

Emerging Contaminants (ECs) (Elorriaga Yanina et al. 2012) are compounds of different origin and chemical nature, which are disseminated in the environment and have been detected in water supply sources, groundwater, wastewater [Stuart et al., 2012] and even in drinking water.

Little is known regarding their presence, impact and treatment; in most cases they are unregulated contaminants, candidates for future regulation, depending on research on their potential health effects and monitoring data regarding their incidence.

These are pesticides, pharmaceuticals, illicit drugs, "lifestyle" compounds, personal care products (PPCPs: Pharmaceuticals and Personal Care Products) and others. The first subgroup (Pharmaceuticals - P) corresponds to the pharmaceuticals themselves, natural or synthetic, used in human and animal therapeutics. The second group includes products for personal use (Personal Care Products - PCPs), whose formulations are based on multifunctional synthesis products (hair dyes, lipsticks, hair gels, cosmetics, shampoos, toothpastes, fragrances, antiperspirants, deodorants, body lotions and creams, bath salts, incense, sunscreens, etc.).

They can be found in solid waste (e.g., urban open-air dumps), urban effluents (domestic, municipal, industrial) or agricultural effluents; activities associated with intensive livestock production (dairy farms, feedlots) or aquaculture also contribute to the environmental dispersion of these pollutants that are eventually incorporated into aquatic, surface or subway environments [Teijón et al., 2010].

Technological advances, particularly in analytical techniques, have contributed to the unequivocal confirmation of their presence, even in trace concentrations, and their quantity in aquatic environments is expanding rapidly. Both in the liquid phases of aquatic environments (surface and subterranean) and in the associated solid phases (sediments), an important diversity of ECs has been detected.

The available evidence shows that the chemical varieties and quantities of these products that are discharged into aquatic environments are steadily increasing.

The complex and varied problems that these pollutants can cause in aquatic environments are associated, among other factors, with their chemical diversity, the inability of the environment to degrade them and the chemical interactions that arise in the environment where they enter, i.e. the combination with other molecules.

The literature [Garcia-Gomez et al., 2011; Teijón et al., 2010; Ferrari et al., 2003] reports that conventional mitigation treatments of liquid effluents (industrial and domestic) prior to their discharge into surface water bodies, which can be vehicles for these products, are not sufficient to retain, degrade or inactivate them prior to their entry into the natural aquatic environments that are their final receptors.

Finally, there is agreement that the concentrations that CEs can reach, particularly in peri-urban water bodies, should be monitored both for their localized or distant adverse effects, with risks to human, plant and animal health [Carrión Cruz 2016; Delgado de Bravo 1996; Di Pace 1992; García Gómez et al. 2011].

1.5 Active Pharmaceutical Ingredients in the aquatic environment [Rebollo et al, 2010].

The aquatic environment has been greatly affected by residues from pharmaceutical compounds [Barceló and López 2007]. These not only affect the biological processes used for the treatment of municipal wastewater, but also exceed the limits of potabilization.

Drug contamination is fundamentally related to the use in urban environments and comes from the endosomatic and exosomatic metabolism of a city [Delgado de Bravo 1996; Di Pace 1992; Duran 1995], it is related to the excretion of drugs or metabolites in urine and feces and the elimination of expired or unconsumed drugs, which continuously enter an aquatic body, in low concentrations, measured in river water in micrograms per liter (contaminant load), which implies that the life cycle of drugs has not been closed and that the reduction of use based on criteria of rationality is fundamental.

The routes of entry of drugs into the environment are: domestic and industrial wastewater (through urine and feces of the patient), hospital effluents (being eliminated through toilets and sinks), effluents from agricultural and livestock activities, septic tanks, etc., as well as from the environment.

MEDICAMENTO Y COMUNIDAD
REGISTRO
COMERCIALIZACION
DISTRIBUCION
PRESCRICCION
DISPENSACION
USO
CADENA DEL MEDICAMENTO
Industria Farmacéutica, Políticos, Reguladores, Gestores de los Sist. de atención de Salud, Inst. Universitarias, Sociedades Científicas, Profesionales de Salud, usuarios, Organizaciones de Consumidores, etc.

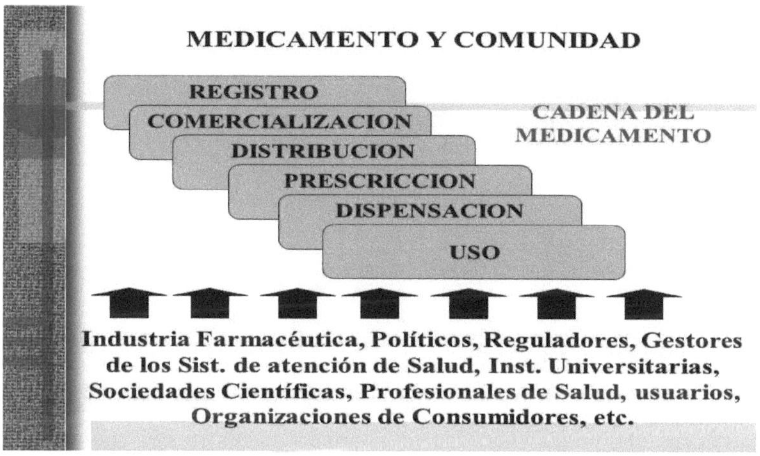

Figure 1 Drug and Community: Drug Chain. [Laporte J.R, Tognioni G. Principles of Drug Epidemiology.2nd Edition].

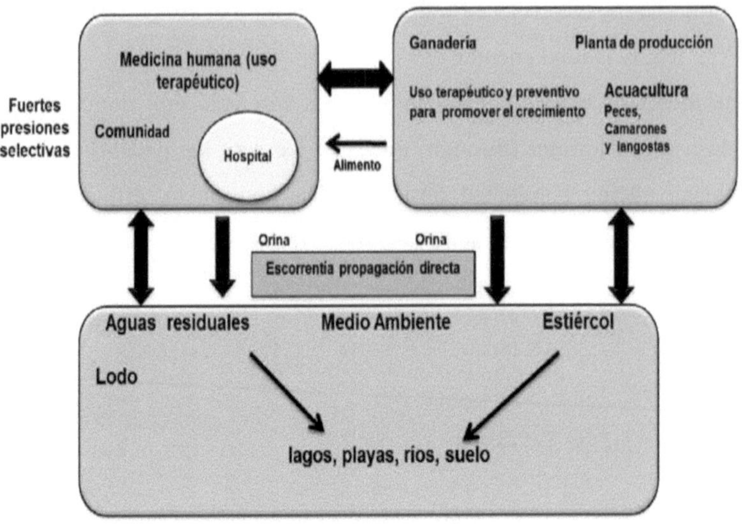

Figure 2 Urban Ecosystem - Natural Environment Interaction (Source: https://www.tecnoaqua.es)

Of all the emerging pollutants, the ones that have probably raised most concern and study in recent years are drugs [Fent et al. 2006] and, in particular, antibiotics. The use of pharmaceuticals in EU countries is estimated in tons per year, and many of the most widely used are antibiotics, which are used in quantities similar to those of pesticides.

As a result of the research carried out so far, some drugs are being considered by the European Union as possible candidates to be included in the list of priority organic pollutants in drinking water; for the time being, no maximum limits have been set for drinking water, but they will most likely be regulated in the near future.

Currently in Europe there are more than 3000 active ingredients permitted for use in health care. However, since the first clofibric acid residue was detected to date, only about 100 of them have ever been analyzed in different environmental compartments [Fatta-Kassinos et al.]

The need to continue working in this line of research, which should include the study of metabolites [Celiz et al., 2009] and transformation products is therefore evident, in addition to the fact that these molecules are continuously entering the environment.

At the moment, the number of articles dedicated to the analysis of drugs in water is much higher than that of the analysis in solid matrices. This is probably due to the great complexity of the study of such matrices. However, technological advances in the field of analytical chemistry make it possible to face this challenge with a high probability of success.

The groups of drugs that are currently considered the most dangerous and require research are: [Ferrari et al, 2004].

-Analgesics: They are one of the most widely consumed drugs worldwide and are considered the most self-medicated (ASHP); diclofenac and ASA were reported to be present in wastewater [Jimenez C 2011], naproxen, ibuprofen and acetaminophen were reported in hospital wastewater. Similarly, the presence of metabolites of ibuprofen has been reported [Celiz et al. 2009]; this is an important indicator of the need to know the metabolic pathways of each of the compounds, to determine or rule out the origin of their toxicity. The persistence in the aquatic environment of drugs such as ibuprofen, diclofenac, carbamazepine, or clofibric acid, which are still present in drinking water, has been of greater concern.

-Antibiotics: These drugs are widely used in the world; their effect against pathogenic microorganisms in animals and humans, as well as their use for food preservation, have increased their production and consumption, allowing large discharges into water bodies [Watkinson et al. 2009] with manifestations of microbial resistance in the study areas. Among the antibiotics most commonly reported in water bodies are tetracyclines, aminoglycosides, macrolides, beta-lactams and vancomycin, among others, with the possibility of the development of resistant bacterial strains that render these compounds ineffective for the therapeutic purpose for which they were designed [Díaz-Cruz et al, 2003] (antibiotics rank third in volume of use of all drugs used in human medicine, and also represent one of the most used in veterinary medicine).

-Antihypertensives: Arterial hypertension, the most common cardiovascular disease in the world. They constitute a very broad group and among them calcium antagonists, angiotensin-converting enzyme inhibitors and beta-blockers, among others, stand out. Some β-blockers such as atenolol, metoprolol and propranolol have reached levels above 0.017μg/L in municipal water effluents.

Contrast media: in X-rays, because they are very persistent, are not removed in treatment plants, and easily reach groundwater by percolation through soils.

-Cytostatics: because due to their high pharmacological potency, they frequently exhibit carcinogenic, mutagenic or embryogenic properties, and, like the previous ones, they appear to show negligible elimination in clearance processes.

-Estrogens: used primarily as contraceptives and for the treatment of hormonal disorders, which are responsible in many cases for the appearance of feminization phenomena, hermaphroditism, and decreased fertility.

It should be remembered that the lists of drugs include several categories of drugs (such as vitamins, electrolytes, amino acids, peptides, carbohydrates, vaccines) that are considered safe. Not all chemicals are contaminants. Not all contaminants are man-made.

1.6 Pharmacokinesis of Chemical Contaminants (IFA)

The kinesis and dynamism of these molecules depends not only on the characteristics of the drug, but also on the matrices of these environments.

Therefore, in order to approach these studies, the temporal and spatial variations of the environment must be considered, with different biodegradation capacities, where CEs can interrupt this process of inactivation of organic matter in the aquatic system.

A realistic assessment of IFAs in the aquatic environment requires an integrated groundwater-soil/sediment-surface water study. The concentrations found in surface water (as a consequence of incomplete removal in water treatment plants) or groundwater (due to the low attenuation of some compounds during percolation through soils) are usually in the range of ng/L or µg/L, while in soils and sediments, where they can persist for long periods of time (the half-life of clofibric acid, for example, is estimated at 21 years), they reach concentrations of up to g/L [Barceló and López, 2007; Barcelo 2008].

An added problem is that their behavior in the environment may be different from that observed in animal and human studies due to different conditions.

Spanish expert Damiá Barceló explains the hazardousness of emerging pollutants by considering the following kinetic and dynamic parameters:

- Persistence: is related to the physicochemical properties of the molecules. Their persistence is expressed by a long half-life due to the fact that they are difficult to degrade, which is a cause for concern, e.g. contrast agents: almost all are organic iodinated compounds, very difficult to degrade photochemically, biologically and/or chemically; hormones that degrade very slowly in the environment, so they can accumulate in the food chain, due to their relative insolubility in water and high solubility in fats; the antibiotic erythromycin, the anti-inflammatory naproxen and the antilipemic clofibric acid will remain unchanged for several years after discharge, but other times, it is their metabolites that are the most persistent.

- Transformations: In water they can be metabolized by oxidation, hydrolysis or photolysis or interact with other molecules, causing hazardous substances to be transformed into potentially more toxic ones, many of them, being biologically active act as endocrine disruptors.

- Bioconcentration: if the substance has more affinity with the tissues than with water, it can reach higher concentrations in the tissues.

- Bioaccumulation: Refers to the net accumulation over time in an organism from both biotic (other organisms) and abiotic (soil, air, water) sources. Many pollutants that are diluted in the medium can magnify their concentration within the cells of organisms reaching high levels of danger. Because the concentration of substances increases with time, older organisms have higher concentrations.

- Biomagnification: It occurs at the ecosystem level, by increasing concentration as it moves up the trophic chain. Biomagnification is a process of bioaccumulation of a toxic substance (e.g. DDT pesticide), which occurs in low concentrations in organisms at the beginning of the food chain and in greater proportion as one moves up the food chain. Biological magnification is the tendency of contaminants to concentrate at successive trophic levels. This is very often to the detriment of the organisms in which these materials are concentrated, as the pollutants are almost always toxic. The concentration of the product in the consuming organism is higher than the concentration of the same product in the consumed organism.

- Environmental mobility: ability to move in the environment. Contaminated water spreads the toxicant to biota, flora and fauna, causing the death of species, an increase in subclinical intoxication in human groups, as well as the loss of water as a usable resource and the probable contamination of aquifers. The factors that control the mobility of contaminants are:- chemical characteristics of the contaminant;- chemical characteristics of the matrix with which the contaminant interacts; physical and biological nature of the environment in which the contaminant will lodge;- physical forces that mobilize the elements in the environment, winds, the flow of a river and physical and chemical processes mediated by the biota.

1.7 Pharmacodynamics of Chemical Contaminants (IFA)

The harmful or undesired consequences associated with drugs in environmental compartments can manifest themselves even when they are found in very low concentrations (organic micropollutants), or in the absence of the molecules that caused them. Their effects on a natural eco-system can be wide-ranging, affecting individuals, populations and communities:

Lethal Effects: Toxicity due to negative effects on animal and plant health. Contaminants can modify the functioning of the trophic chain, breaking food relationships between producers, consumers and decomposers. In a trophic chain, each link (trophic level) obtains the energy necessary for life from the immediately preceding level; in this way, energy flows through the chain in a linear and ascending manner.

It should be noted that a high rate of environmental degradation does not ensure the subsequent toxicological safety of a drug in the aquatic environment, since the transformation products generated may also exhibit toxicity or be bioaccumulated by other species co-inhabiting the same site. By damaging the functioning of the trophic chain, chemical pollutants generate a crisis in biodiversity.

A food chain, strictly speaking, has several disadvantages if a link disappears: -The link that depends directly on it will disappear with it, since it will be left without food and without the energy necessary to sustain itself; the level that loses its predators will be overpopulated, the lower levels and the contiguous levels will be unbalanced, due to the lack of competition between that species and the one that makes up the missing link.

Biodiversity loss is the result of a process of deterioration of natural ecosystems, which is characteristic of the current environmental crisis.

An example of this situation is the case of diclofenac, which, apart from affecting the kidneys in mammals, has been associated (as a consequence of its use in veterinary medicine) with the disappearance of white vultures in India and Pakistan, which, according to the author of this study [Fent K et al, 2006], is an ecological disaster comparable to what happened in the past with DDT. Another example is that of propanolol, which Dr. Barceló's research team has detected on multiple occasions in Spain, and which has been shown to have harmful effects on zooplankton as well as on benthic organisms. [Fent K et al., 2006].

Sublethal effects: although they may appear to be less dangerous than lethal effects, they are greater in the population and may be manifested by modifications at the genetic, biochemical, physiological, behavioral or life cycle levels. Sub-lethal effects are not easy to identify. The use of biochemical biomarkers has allowed progress to be made in identifying them.

The most serious environmental effects are seen for endocrine disrupting compounds (Argemi, F2005) (Fernandez, M 2014) with claims that exposure to sewage treatment plants can cause feminization in some fish species: contraceptive estrogens have had this effect in several fish and amphibian species. The hormones are considered toxic to algae, invertebrates and fish. They greatly affect fish that readily absorb them and modify their reproductive process and even their sexual behavior. Organisms exposed to more than one pollutant may present additive, antagonistic or synergistic toxic effects, thus the effects may be null, lethal or sublethal.

Mutations: Antineoplastics are normally found in liquid effluents, they are drugs that take quite a long time to be eliminated by the human organism. The highest concentrations are detected in hospital effluents. They are dangerous because they are considered mutagenic and toxic for reproduction. They are not well eliminated in sewage treatment plants and are very persistent in the environment as they are poorly biodegradable. The effects manifest themselves more frequently in the offspring than in the exposed parent. Bacterial Resistance: The use and abuse of antibiotics means that they are found in a very high level in the liquid effluents of hospitals and urban centers. Some antibiotics are degraded in wastewater treatment plants but others are not and are reintroduced into the environment. They are found with some frequency in the drinking water distributed. Antibiotics disrupt the natural bacterial community and contribute to an increase in resistant bacteria. Man can thus ingest antibiotic residues, not only through drinking water, but also by eating fish and shellfish, disrupting the normal intestinal flora.

1.8 Bibliography

Argemi, F; Cianini, N; Porta, A. Endocrine Disruption Environmental Perspectives and Public Health. Acta Bioquim. Clin Latinoam 39, 3 (2005).

Barceló D. and López MJ. (2007). Contamination and chemical quality of water: the problem of emerging pollutants. Scientific-Technical Panel for monitoring water policy. Institute of Chemical and Environmental Research-CSIC. Barcelona.

Barceló D. (2008). Consejo Superior de Investigaciones Científicas (Spain), editors. Aguas continentales. Madrid: Consejo Superior de Investigaciones Científicas. 276 p. (CSIS Reports).

Carrión Cruz D.A. (2014). Wastewater treatment and its influence on the right to a healthy environment of citizens living in the environment of the Machángara river south of the Metropolitan District of Quito. [B.S. Thesis].

Cattogio J. (1993). Contaminantes ambientales, Material de estudio Especialidad Ambiente y Patología Ambiental, Escuela de Patología Ambiental, Facultad de Medicina, UNP, S/P.

Celiz M.D., Tso J., Aga D.S. (2009). Pharmaceutical metabolites in the environment: analytical challenges and ecological risks. Environ Toxicol Chem 28, 2473-2484.

Dhillon G., Kaur S., Pulicharla R., Brar S., Cledon M., Verma M., Surampalli RY. (2015). Triclosan: Current Status, Occurrence, Environmental Risks and Bioaccumulation Potential. Int J Environ Res Public Health. 12(5), 5657-5684.

Delgado de Bravo, M. Ambiente y Calidad de vida: una respuesta a los problemas de las metrópolis latinoamericanas, Buenos Aires 1996.

Dictionary of the Royal Spanish Academy (Twenty-second Edition).

Díaz-Cruz M.S., López de Alda M.J., Barcelo D. (2003). Environmental behavior and analysis of veterinary and human drugs in soils, sediments and sludge. Trends in Analytical Chemistry, Vol. 22 (6), 340-351.

Di Pace M., Feoeaovisky S. Haadoy J., Mazzucchelli S. (1992). Urban Environment in Argentina, Buenos Aires. CEAL.

Duran D., Baxendale C.,Bortagaray L.,Buzai G., Casas R., Curto de Casas S., Fuschini Mejias M.,Paso Viola L.,Pierre L., Roccatagliata J. Torchio M. (1995) La Argentina ambiental: Naturaleza y sociedad. Buenos Aires.

Elorriaga Y., Marino D.J., Carriquiriborde P., Ronco A.E. (2012). Emerging contaminants. Pharmaceuticals in the environment. 7th Environmental Congress. UNLP. Available at: http://www.congresos.unlp.edu.ar/index.php/CCMA/7CCMA/paper/viewFile/932/216.

Fatta-Kassinos D., Meric S., Nicolaou A. (2011). Pharmaceutical residues in environmental waters and wastewater: current state of knowledge and future research. Anal Bioanal Chem 399, 251-275.

Ferrari B., Mons R., Vollat B., Fraysse B., Lo Giudice R., Pollio A. and Garric J. (2004). Environmental risk assessment of six human pharmaceuticals Are the current environmental risk assessment procedures sufficient for the protection of the aquatic environment? Environmental Toxicology and chemistry 23 (5), 1344-54.

Fent K., Weston A. and Caminada D. (2006). Ecotoxicology of human pharmaceuticals. In: Aquat Toxicol. 76, 122-59.

Fernández M and Olea N. Endocrine Disruptors, enough evidence to act? Instituto de Investigación Biosanitaria de Granada,University of Granada; CIBER de Epidemiología y Salud Pública, CIBERESP, Spain. Gac Sanit.2014; 28(2): 93-95.

García-Gómez C., Gortáres-Moroyoqui P., Drogui P. (2011). Emerging contaminants: effects and removal treatments Emerging contaminants: effects and removal treatments. Rev Quimica Viva 10(2), 96-105.

Halden UK. 2015. Epistemology of contaminants of emerging concern and literature meta-analysis. J Hazard Mater 282, 2-9.

Jiménez C. (2011). Emerging organic contaminants in the environment: pharmaceuticals. Rev. Lasallista Investig. 8 (2), 143-153.

Rebollo C., Gros Calvo M., Lopez M., Petrovic A., Ginebrada Marti A., Barceló Culleres D. (2011). "Sanitary repercussions of water quality: drug residues in water". Rev. salud ambient. 11(1-2), 17-26.

Sánchez E. (2002). The precautionary principle: implications for public health. Gac Sanit., 16(5), 371-3.

Stuart M. Lapworth D., Crane E., Hart A. (2012). Review of risk from potential emerging contaminants in UK groundwater. Science of the Total Environment 416, 1-21.

Teijon G., Candela L., Tamoh K., Molina-Díaz A., Fernández-Alba A.R. (2010). Occurrence of emerging contaminants, priority substances (2008/105/CE) and heavy metals in treated wastewater and groundwater at Depurbaix facility (Barcelona, Spain). Science of the Total Environment 408, 3584-3595.

Watkinson A.J., Murby E.J., Kolpin D.W., Costanzo S.D. (2009). The occurrence of antibiotics in an urban water shed: From waste water to drinking water. Sci Total Environ. 407, 2711-2723.

Chapter 2

History of Pharmaco-contamination

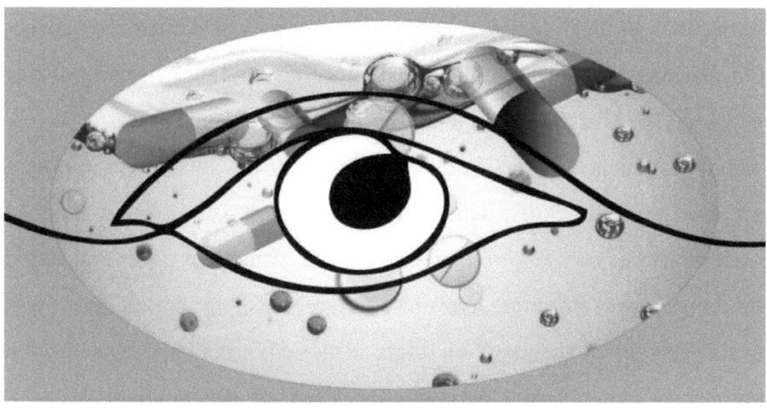

2.1 Urban River Pollution: Emerging Contaminants
2.2 Aquaterra - Model Key projects in Spanish rivers
2.3 Pharmaco-pollution in other rivers in Europe and the world
2.4 Bibliography

2.1 Urban River Pollution - Emerging Contaminants

Human activity is increasing the pressure on ecosystems, which leads to drastic changes, since they are not isolated in nature and, due to their interaction, produce network effects that are not immediately perceived, thus causing problems that are apparently local and that, because of this network effect, become a regional problem [Barragán 2011].

The first evidence of the presence of drugs in the aquatic environment occurred in the 1970s with the identification of clofibric acid in wastewater in the USA, which is the active metabolite of several blood lipid regulators (clofibrate, etofilin clofibrate, and etofibrate), and it was in the 1990s that the issue of drugs in the environment began to gain momentum, mainly in 1998 with the work of Rapport and the eco-systemic approach to health [Rapport et al. 2000].

In addition to agro-industrial pollution of ecosystems, pollution of urban origin, chemical pollutants from personal care products, various activities and drug residues, known as Emerging Pollutants [Daughton and Ternes, 1999 - Jjemba 2006 - Barceló 2007].

Urban chemical contaminants originate in occupational settings, among them are pharmaceutical wastes [Jimenez 2011] (active pharmaceutical ingredients) which are eliminated from sanitary settings [Kummerer 2001] and also domiciliary [Bound et al., 2006] reaching the environment through sewage.

The search for emerging chemical contaminants, is performed in wastewater [Kummerer 2009- Fatta-Kassinos et al., 2011-Wang and Wang 2016] afferent and efferent from WWTPs [Aznar 2016], in river surface water, in and groundwater [Sui et al., 2015] and sediments [Hernando et al., 2006].

2.2 Aquaterra Project - Model Key Project

The monitoring of drugs and drugs of abuse carried out by the Department of Environmental Chemistry, Institute of Environmental Diagnosis (Barceló D 2008) and Water Studies (IDAEA); Consejo Superior de Investigaciones Científicas (CSIC) [Barceló 2008] Institut Catalá de Recerca de l' Aigua (ICRA) and Institució Catalana de Reserca i Estudis Avancats (ICREA) constitute the strongest scientific evidence. They were carried out in the aquatic environment of the Llobregat and Ebro river basins, in order to evaluate water quality in relation to the presence of these substances. These works are financed with the help of the European projects AQUATERA and MODEL KEY (2005).

The Aquaterra project of the Instituto de Investigaciones Químicas y Ambientales del Consejo Superior de Investigaciones Científicas de España (CSIC) gave the alert in 2005, after analyzing the waters of five rivers in Europe, among them the Ebro, with a screening in 18 points along the river, being all positive. Dozens of drugs belonging to different pharmacological groups that act on the CNS were found: psychotropics (diazepam); antiepileptics (carbamazepine); on the CV apparatus: beta blockers (atenolol, propanolol); cholesterol regulators (bezafibrate); antibiotics: amoxicillin, sulfamethoxazole; analgesics: ibuprofen, diclofenac; contraceptives; steroids; contrast media.

The danger of the Network Effect is expressed when pharmaceutical compounds were identified downstream of the discharge point of the urban sewage treatment plants as the main source of emission of these pollutants into the aquatic environment; the profile of contamination by pharmaceuticals being quite similar in the rivers studied.

In addition to the identification of the drugs, the reports include concentration and environmental risk indexes (HQ) calculated for the drugs at different trophic levels (algae, daphnids, fish); they indicate that the compounds with the highest eco-toxicological risk in the Llobregat are sulfamethoxazole for algae, gemfibrosil for algae and fish, clofibric acid and erythromycin for daphnids, ibuprofen for all trophic links. In the Ebro, the most problematic compounds are sulfamethoxazole for algae, erythromycin, clofibric acid and fluoxetine for daphnids.

The presence of antibiotics and the danger of the emergence of bacterial resistance [Watkinson et al., 2009, Kummerer 2004, Dang et al., 2007] with its serious pharmacotherapeutic consequences, shows the need to restore the health of eco-systems; pharmaceutical residues are toxic to the ecosystem [Fent et al., 2006; -Sanderson et al., 2003], affecting the life of the ecosystem, with the danger to humans of inadvertent exposure [Daughton 2008].

The discharge of antibiotics damages the environment by causing toxic effects. In a study by the Autonomous University of Madrid (UAM) and the University of Alcalá published in the journal "Water Research", mixtures of antibiotics from different families increase the risk of toxicity, even when the concentrations are low, leading to a synergistic effect, affecting cyanobacteria and green algae, primary producers of eco-systems, according to the signatory of the work Francisca Fernadez Piñas, those detected were: amoxicillin, erythromycin, quinolones, tetracyclines. Erythromycin is a compound toxic to green algae and cyanobacteria to such an extent that it can be labeled under EU regulations as very toxic to aquatic life. A risk quotient was also calculated, which is the ratio between the concentration measured in the environment and the concentration at which it does not represent a risk; concentrations greater than unity indicate concentrations that are harmful to organisms in the environment. Several pharmacological groups have already been identified in the aquatic environment, hypolipidemic agents to which clofibric acid belongs, although it was one of the first to be detected, are still present in the environment [Emblidge and DeLorenze, 2006]; the presence of synthetic steroids [Aherne and Briggs 1989], the presence of estrogens in wastewater and surface water [Sole et al, 2000] accompany its discovery. The Llobregat river basin was the first Spanish basin in which the existence of effects on the biota expressed by feminization phenomena in fish, caused by the presence of endocrine disruptors with estrogenic activity and the existence of intersex fish (fish with simultaneous male and female reproductive organs), was revealed.

This worrying finding occurred in the course of a monitoring program carried out between 1999 and 2002, in which the levels of estrogens and alkylphenol-type detergents, ethoxylated, measured in water and sediments in two of the main tributaries of the Llobregat were elevated. The effects were evidenced by the presence of abnormally high concentrations of plasma vitellogenin in carp (vitellogenin is an egg yolk precursor protein used as an indicator of exposure to estrogenic compounds).

Numerous published articles aroused great scientific and social interest at the time (as occurred in Spain after the publication in the press of some of the results obtained by Dr. Barceló's research team: El Periódico, 26 October 2005; El País, 17 January 2006; El global, 30 January 2006).

In 2010 in the Ebro basin, 77 compounds, including drugs and active metabolites, were analyzed after discharge from wastewater treatment plants. For this purpose they sampled in 24 areas of different locations; the following drugs were found in all of them: analgesics, antiepileptic, antibiotics, β-blocker, antineoplastic. Analgesics and anti-inflammatory drugs, such as Ibuprofen, Diclofenac and Mefenamic Acid, were eliminated by more than 80%, however others were eliminated little or not at all as was the case with the anti-epileptic Carbamazepine, macrolide antibiotics and Trimetroprime. Works with clear methodology showing the limitation of the purification plants to eliminate the pharmaceutical pollutant compounds, the elimination of them was not adequate.

Estimates made within the framework of the AQUATERRA project indicate that pesticides used for the cultivation of vines and corn have an annual load in the Ebro river of 800 to 500 kg respectively; the same type of calculation applied to the drugs most commonly found in the Ebro river, such as Paracetamol, Ibuprofen, Carbamazepine and Atenolol, indicate that approximately 100 kg of each of these drugs are discharged into the river after passing through the treatment stations in the whole basin. In total, about 30 drugs have been monitored, which represents about 3000 kg per year or 3 tons of drugs. This quantity is the one that finally reaches the river, since the load entering the WWTP treatment stations is about 5 times higher.

In the same year 2010, in the Llobregat river, effluents from conventional municipal wastewater treatment plants were also compared with those resulting from additional tertiary treatment, using ultrafiltration, reverse osmosis and UV treatment, and the aquifer was also analyzed. In the effluents from the conventional treatment they found average values above 1000 μg/L of Atenolol (β-blocker), Diclofenac (anti-inflammatory), Furosemide and Hydrochlorothiazide (diuretics), Gemfibrozil (lipid regulator) and two metabolites of the analgesic metamizole. If tertiary treatment was performed, the values decreased to around 100 μg/L, i.e., they were an order of magnitude lower, although they found that only a small number of compounds, of the 170 studied, were completely eliminated with tertiary treatment. Regarding the concentration levels, it was found that the flow of the Ebro had a dilution effect and lowered the levels, reaching concentrations of the order of ng/L.

The evaluation of the environmental risk in Spanish rivers caused by emerging pollutants shows that there is a real urban chemical soup in them, to which inorganic pollutants such as heavy metals are added, making it necessary to reduce the presence of pollutants and their environmental impact [Ginebreda et al. 2010; EEA 2010; Roig 2010].

2.3 Pharmaco-pollution in other rivers in Europe and the world.

There are numerous antecedents of urban drug-pollution of rivers in different continents, thus being a worldwide problem for the sustainable development of the environment [WHO/PAHO 2000].

In Sweden, a study was carried out in 2005 on the presence of antibiotics in effluents: Norfloxacin, Ofloxacin, Ciprofloxacin, Doxycycline, Sulfamethoxazole and Trimethoprim. This study shows the presence of drugs not only in the river water, but also in the mud. The antibiotics norfloxacin, ofloxacin, ciprofloxacin, were the most detected in the sludge, with levels of mg /Kg of dry sample. Some studies have shown that when sludge is applied to soils there is greater persistence of antibiotics than in aquatic environments, due to the fact that their adsorption to the soil decreases their availability for biodegradation.

In 2006, the first Environmental Impact Assessment Guide [Guia 2006] was published, initiating the search for and identification of several therapeutic classes of drugs by chromatography and spectrometry of hospital effluents and problematic aquatic streams [Gómez et al. 2006; Richardson 2009].

A group of drugs that have been widely studied are the anti-inflammatory drugs that affect aquatic and terrestrial biota. A study in Asia in 2010 showed that Diclofenac had been the cause of death of millions of vultures on that continent. The drug had been widely used as a medicine for sick livestock, especially cows, which were left in the field when they died and served as food for scavenger birds. Diclofenac caused acute renal failure in the birds and they died within a few days. The result was the almost total disappearance (97%) of three species of vultures, which are now in danger of extinction. This example, although it does not occur in an aquatic environment, shows the effects of the contaminant at the biological and environmental level on biodiversity.

The potential effects of contaminants on humans require further research, since not only active pharmaceutical ingredients are involved, but also their metabolites [Celiz et al, 2009], which maintain the capacity to generate biological changes.

In addition to the search for biologically active molecules, environmental studies in problem rivers show temporal variations in chemical contamination [Veach and Bernot 2011], as a result of the dilution effect of aquatic currents.

In Argentina, the VII Environmental Congress was held in La Plata in 2012 [Elorriaga et al., 2012], and pharmacoecovigilance studies were carried out in the Province of Córdoba in the Suquia river [Valdés et al., 2014].

Drugs were detected in the Suquia River in the Province of Córdoba (Valdés et al., 2014) ciprofloxacin, enalapril, estrone, dihydrotestosterone, oxcarbazepine, carbamazepine and diclofenac. The researchers took samples at five points along the Suquia: La Calera (between San Roque Dam and the City of Córdoba), Chacra de la Merced (immediately after Bajo Grande), Villa Corazón de María, Capilla de los Remedios and Rio Primero, 70 km from the wastewater treatment plant. They also collected a sample in the Yuspe River, in the mountainous area and tributary of the Suquia, a pure water course. This study shows that the main source of contamination is the Wastewater Treatment Plant (WWTP) in Bajo Grande, since the IFA are present only in the sites downstream of this plant. The highest concentration was atenolol: 581 nanograms per liter of water in Villa Corazon de Maria. The concentration of this drug and diclofenac was decreasing as samples were taken further away from Bajo Grande. However, 70 km below the WWTP in Rio Primero, the drugs are still present. The river fails to purify these substances. The research was published in Science of the Total Environment and involved scientists from the Clinical Biochemistry and Immunology Research Center (CIBICI), the Institute of Animal Diversity and Ecology (IDEA) and the Institute of Food Science and Technology of Córdoba (ICYTAC).

Works from Chile [Henriquez 2010], from Uruguay [Niell et al. 2013], in wastewater from Montevideo. This Uruguayan work highlights the presence of caffeine, nicotine, paraxanthine, theobromine, carbamazepine, ibuprofen and acetaminophen residues (Niell).

Work from Brazil: In the Atibaia River of São Paulo (Brazil), studies have been conducted for the determination of 15 emerging contaminants in surface waters: acetoaminophenol, salicylic acid, diclofenac, ibuprofen, caffeine, 17 β-estradiol, estrone, progesterone, 17 α-ethinylestradiol, levonorgestrel, diethyl, dibutyl phthalate, 4-Octylphenol, 4-nonylphenol and bisphenol. [Montagner and Jardim 2011]

In 2012 a review of the potential risks of emerging contaminants in river water, including the study of groundwater, also found that carbamazepine was the most frequently detected drug, with a range of maximum values between 40 and 570 ng/L in different countries. While in Switzerland, Austria, Germany, Japan, USA, France, Serbia and Spain, anti-inflammatory and analgesic drugs such as Ibuprofen, Diclofenac and Paracetamol were the most frequently detected.

The anti-inflammatory Ibuprofen [Buser et al., 1999] and Naproxen, also in surface waters, as well as in a comparative study published in 2013 showed the highest concentrations in rivers in the United Kingdom, Canada and Japan at levels of μg/L while in other countries, out of a total of fourteen, they did not exceed pg/L or ng/L, a fact that was related to the different use of these compounds in each country. In these studies, in addition to presence and identification, the contaminant load and its association with the consumption habits of each population are measured.

A review on the presence of antibiotics in aquatic environments in Europe was published in 2016, the authors cite that they have been detected in influents and effluents from wastewater treatment plants (WWTP), rivers, groundwater and drinking water; depending on the antibiotic class and environmental matrix, concentrations ranged from ng/L to several μg/L. In Switzerland, Austria, Germany, Japan, USA, France, Serbia and Spain. Presence and identification in surface water, groundwater and drinking water, quinolones, sulfonamides and trimethoprim are the antibiotics mainly analyzed and detected, due to their importance in human and veterinary medicine and their persistence in the aqueous medium. For example, some fluoroquinolones are excreted up to 70% without being metabolized and this fact could be related to the appearance of microbial resistance; this family of antibiotics has a high affinity for soil, sludge and sediments and a half-life ranging from 10.6 days in surface water to 580 days in soils.

Very low concentrations of these pharmacological compounds were found in drinking water, which is reassuring; however, in the Lisbon drinking water system, water samples collected from the EPAL (Empresa Portuguesa das Águas Livres S.A.) supply system were quantified and the following analytes were found: carbamazepine, atenolol, sulfadiazine, sulfamethazine, sulfapyridine, sulfamethoxazole, paracetamol, caffeine and erythromycin. Presence in drinking water.

A bibliographic study on three compounds has been published in early 2017: an anti-inflammatory Diclofenac, and two hormones, one natural, 17-beta-Estradiol, and another synthetic, 17-alpha-Etinylestradiol; the work has compiled and analyzed information published for twenty years, specifically from 1995 to 2015, and studies both the sources of contamination and the methods of monitoring and control in all European countries. These studies establish the need to build a list of drugs that require monitoring because of their potential risk to the aquatic environment. [European Commission].

From the bibliography analyzed, they selected 1,268 publications, and found that among the European countries that studied the contamination of aquatic environments, Spain had published the largest number of papers, 19.2% (285 publications), followed by Germany, with 16.3%, and then the United Kingdom, with 12%. The remaining countries did not exceed 10% of publications each.

The evaluation of the capacity of the WWTPs to remove the drugs shows that 25-40% of Diclofenac was removed and that the average concentration in the effluent was between 0.002 and 2.5 μg/L; the removal of hormones was higher, in the order of 85% or higher, so that only nanograms per liter remained in the effluent.

The problem of pharmaco-pollution is assumed to be a problem of the European continent, although the presence of emerging contaminants in the environment is not new, their effects on human health and the environment have only recently been studied, unlike in the old continent, in most Latin American countries there are still no adequate legal regulations to regulate them.

In Europe the Parliament Directive (made in 2013) extended the list to 45 priority substances of which 21 are identified as hazardous; which reinforces the need to look for new alternatives for the correct detection and disposal of these substances in both drinking water and wastewater treatment plants.

This justifies the need to build knowledge on emerging pollutants to reduce their environmental impact on the aquatic environment, and the need to eliminate them from water, which motivates the use of various unconventional treatments, which should be applied by sewage treatment plants [Rivera Utrilla et al.] In addition to providing kinetic information: presence, persistence, concentration, pharmacodynamic data, pharmaco-ecovigilance investigations show modifications in the biota of the eco-systems, belonging to animal and plant species.

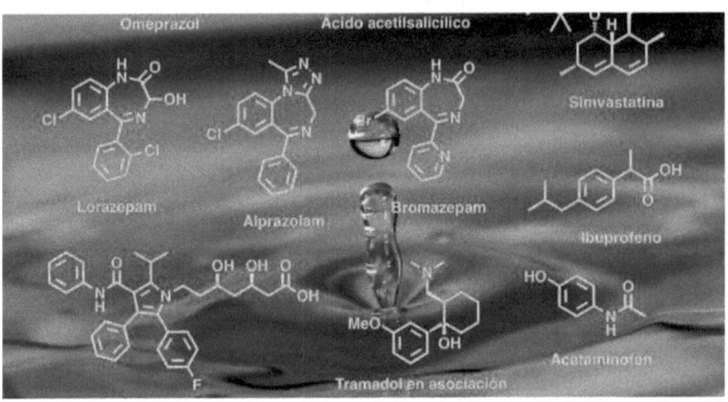

Figure 3 Chemical structures of some pharmaceuticals detected in wastewater (Source: https://www.tecnoaqua.es)

2.4 Bibliography

Aznar R, Albero B, Sánchez-Brunete C, Miguel E, Martín-Girela I, Tadeo JL (2016). Simultaneous determination of multiclass emerging contaminants in aquatic plants by ultrasound-assisted matrix solid-phase dispersion and GC-MS. Environ Sci Pollut 9, 7911-7920.

Aherne GW. and Briggs R. (1989). The relevance of presence of certain synthetic steroids in the aquatic environment. J Pharm Pharmacol 41, 735.

Barceló, D and López, M J. (2007). Contamination and chemical quality of water: the problem of emerging pollutants. Scientific-Technical Panel for monitoring water policy. Institute of Chemical and Environmental Research-CSIC. Barcelona

Barceló D. (2008). Consejo Superior de Investigaciones Científicas (Spain), editors. Continental waters. Madrid: Consejo Superior de Investigaciones Científicas; 276 p. (CSIS Reports).

Barragan J.M. (2011). "Chapter 13. Litorales". Montes, C. (Coord.) Evaluación de los Ecosistemas del Milenio de España. Universidad Autónoma de Madrid, Madrid, pp. 673- 739.

Bound J.P., K. Kitsou and N. Vouvoulis (2006). Household disposal of pharmaceuticals and perception of the risk to the environment. Environmental Toxicology and Pharmacology 21, 301-307.

Buser H.; Poiger T. and Müller M. (1999). Occurrence and environmental behavior of the chiral pharmaceutical drug ibuprofen in surface waters and in wastewater. Environ. Sci. Technol. 33, (15), 2529-2535.

Carrión Cruz DA. (2016). Wastewater treatment and its influence on the right to a healthy environment of citizens living in the environment of the Machángara river south of the Metropolitan District of Quito in 2014. [B.S. thesis]. Quito: UCE.

Celiz MD, Tso J, Aga DS (2009). Pharmaceutical metabolites in the environment: analytical challenges and ecological risks. Environ Toxicol Chem 28, 2473-2484.

Dang H., Zhang X., Song L., Chang Y., Yang G. (2007). Molecular determination of oxytetracycline-resistant bacteria and their resistance genes from mariculture environments of China. In: Journal of applied microbiology 103 (6), 2580-2592.

Daughton CG (2008). Pharmaceuticals as environmental pollutants: the ramifications for human exposure. Internat Encyclopedia Public Health 5, 66-102.

Delgado de Bravo, M. Ambiente y Calidad de vida: una respuesta a los problemas de los metrópolis latinoamericanas, Buenos Aires (1996). 55-
Dictionary of the Royal Spanish Academy (Twenty-second Edition).

Dhillon G.S., Kaur S., Pilicharla R., Kaur Brar S., Cledon M., Verma M., Surampalli R.Y. (2015). Triclosan: Current Status, Occurrence, Environmental Risks and Bioaccumulation Potential. Int. J. Environ. Res. Public Health, 12, 5657-5684.

Díaz-Cruz M.S., López de Alda M.J., Barcelo D. (2003). Environmental behavior and analysis of veterinary and human drugs in soils, sediments and sludge. Trends in Analytical Chemistry, 22 (6), 340-351.

Di Pace M. Sustainable cities: urbanization and the environment in the international Perspective - Chap. 8 "Latin America" Westview Press - N. York - 1992.

Duran, R. La Argentina ambiental, Buenos Aires, 1995.

EEA (European Environment Agency), (2010). Pharmaceuticals in the environment. Results of an EEA workshop. EEA Technical Report No1, 20 pp.

Elorriaga Y., Marino D., Carriquiriborde P., and Ronco A. (2012). Emerging Contaminants: Pharmaceutical products in the environment. VII Environmental Congress. La Plata, Argentina.Available from internet at: http://congresos.unlp.edu.ar/index.php

Emblidge J.P. and M.E. DeLorenze (2006). Preliminary Risk Assessment of the lipid-regulating pharmaceutical clofibric acid, for three estuarine species. Environmental Research 100, 216-226.

Fatta-Kassinos D., Meric S., and Nicolaou A. (2011). Pharmaceutical residues in environmental waters and wastewater: current state of knowledge and future research. Anal Bioanal Chem 399, 251-275.

Fent K., Weston A. and Caminada D. (2006). Ecotoxicology of human pharmaceuticals. Aquat Toxicol. 76, 122-59.

Ferrari B., Paxeus N., Lo Giudice R., Pollio A., Garric J. (2003). Ecotoxicological impact of pharmaceuticals found in treated wastewaters:

study of carbamazepine, clofibric acid, and diclofenac. Ecotoxicol. Environ. Safe. 55(3), 359-370.

Ginebreda A., Muñoz I., López de Alda M., Brix R., Lopez Doval J., Barcelo D. (2010). Environmental risk assessment of pharmaceuticals in rivers: relationships between hazard indexes and aquatic macroinvertebrate diversity indexes in the Llobregat River (NE Spain). Environ Internat 36, 153-162

Gaffney V de J., Cardoso VV., Rodrigues A., Ferreira E., Benoliel MJ. and Almeida CM. (2014). Analysis of pharmaceutical compounds in water by SPE-UPLC-ESI-MS/MS. Quím Nova. 37(1),138-149.

García-Gómez C.; Gortáres-Moroyoqui P., Drogui P. (2011). Emerging contaminants: effects and removal treatments Química Viva 10 (2), 96-105.

Gómez M. (2006). Determination of pharmaceuticals of various therapeutic classes by solid-phase extraction and liquid chromatography-tandem mass spectrometry analysis in hospital effluent wastewaters. In: Journal of Chromatography. A. 1114 (2), 224-233.

Guidance for the environmental impact assessment of medicinal products for human use by the EMA (2006) (EMEA/CHMP/SWP/4447/00 corr1) Accessed November 4, 2016.

Hernando M.D., Mezcua M., Fernández-Alba A.R., and Barceló D. (2006). Environmental risk assessment of pharmaceutical residues in wastewater effluents, surface waters and sediments. Talanta 69, 334-342.

Henríquez D. (2010). Presence of emerging contaminants in water and their impact on the ecosystem. Case study: pharmaceutical products in the Biobío river basin, Biobío region, Chile. Thesis, Santiago de Chile.

Jjemba PK (2006). Excretion and ecotoxicity of pharmaceutical and personal care products in the environment. Ecotoxicol Environ Saf 63, 113-130.

Jiménez, C. (2011). Emerging organic pollutants in the environment: pharmaceuticals. In: Rev. Lasallista Investig. 8 (2), 143-153.

Montagner CC. and Jardim WF. (2011). Spatial and seasonal variations of pharmaceuticals and endocrine disruptors in the Atibaia River, São Paulo State (Brazil).J Braz Chem Soc. 22(8), 1452-1462.

Niell S., Colazzo M., Besil N., Cesio V. and Heinzen H. Preliminary evaluation of the occurrence of emerging contaminants in wastewater from Montevideo, Uruguay. In: VII Environmental Congress [Internet]. 2013 [cited 2016 July 8]. Available from: http://sedici.unlp.edu.ar/handle/10915/26665

Kümmerer K. (2001). Drugs in the environment: emission of drugs, diagnostic aids and disinfectants into wastewater by hospitals in relation to other sources da review. In: Chemosphere. 45, 957-969.

Kümmerer K. (2004). Resistance in the environment. Journal of Antimicrobial Chemotherapy 54, 311-320.

Kümmerer K. (2009). The presence of pharmaceuticals in the environment due to human use present knowledge and future challenges. Journal of Environmental Management 90, 2354-2366.

Rapport D., Hildén M., Weppling K., (2000). Restoring the health of the earth's ecosystems: A new challenge for the earth sciences. Episodes, 23(1), 12-19.

Richardson S. (2009). Water analysis: emerging contaminants and current issues. Anal. Chem. 81(12), 4645-4677.

Rivera-Utrilla J., Sánchez-Polo M., Ferro-García MA., Prados-Joya G. and Ocampo Perz R. (2013). Pharmaceuticals as emerging contaminants and their removal from water. A review. Chemosphere 93, 1268-1287.

Roig B. (Editor) (2010). Pharmaceuticals in the environment: current knowledge and need assessment to reduce presence and impact. IWA Publishing, London

Sanderson H, Johnson DJ, Wilson CJ, Brain RA. and Solomon KR. (2003). Probabilistic Hazard assessment of environmentally occurring pharmaceuticals toxicity to fish, daphnids and algae by ECOSAR screening Toxicology Letters 144(3), 383-9.

Sole M., Lopez de Alda MJ., Castillo M., Porte C., Ladegaard-Pedersen K. and Barceló D. (2000). Estrogenicity determination in sewage treatment plants and surface wáters from. The Catalonian area (NE Spain). Environt Sci Technol 34, 5076-5083.

Stuart M., Lapworth D., Crane E., and Hart A. (2012). Review of risk from potential emerging contaminants in UK groundwater. Sci Total Environ., 416, 1-21.

Sui Q., Cao X., Lu S., Zhao W., Qiu Z., and Yu G. (2015). Occurrence, sources and fate of pharmaceuticals and personal care products in the groundwater: A review. Emerging Contaminants 1, 14-24.

Teijon G., Candela L., Tamoh K., Molina Díaz A. and Fernández-Alba A.R. (2010). Occurrence of emerging contaminants, priority substances (2008/105/CE) and heavy metals in treated wastewater and groundwater at Depurbaix. Science of the Total Environment 408, 3584- 3595.

Valdés ME, Amé MV, Bistoni MDLA, Wunderlin DA (2014). Occurrence and bioaccumulation of pharmaceuticals in a fish species inhabiting the Suquía River basin (Córdoba, Argentina). Sci Total Environ. 472, 389-396.

Veach AM and Bernot MJ (2011). Temporal variation of pharmaceuticals in an urban and agriculturally influenced stream. Sc Total Environ 409, 4553-4563.

Wang J and Wang S (2016). Removal of pharmaceuticals and personal care products (PPCPs) from wastewater: A review.... Journal of Environmental Management 182, 620-640.

Watkinson A.J., Murbyd E.J., Kolpine D.W., Costanzo S.D. (2009). The occurrence of antibiotics in an urban water shed: From waste water to drinking water. In: Sci Total Environ. 407, 2711-2723.

Chapter 3

Resilience of a Freshwater Eco-system

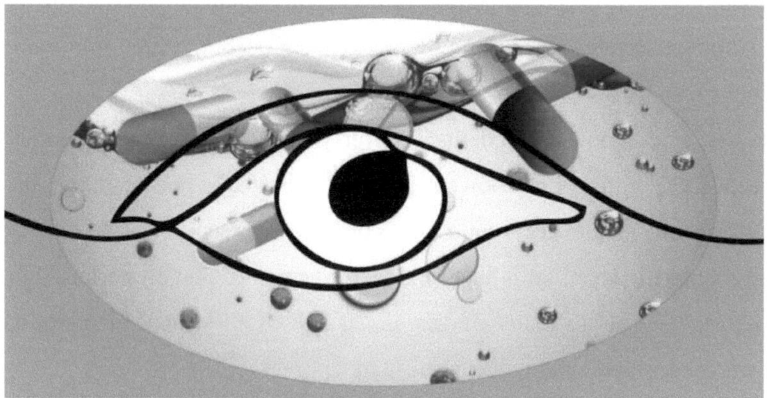

3.1 Purification in freshwater streams.
3.2 Zones in a self-purifying stream
3.3 Role of oxygen in self-purification
3.4 Parameters for measuring Self-Purification
3.5 Self-purification of emerging contaminants
3.6 Bibliography

3.1 Purification in freshwater streams.

Self-purification is the natural resilience of a watercourse, in the face of a pollution process, to recover the physicochemical and biological conditions prior to discharge. The pollutants are diluted in the water body and progressively transformed by biochemical decomposition into more stable forms.

It has long been observed that a river polluted by sewage gradually recovers its initial purity downstream of the discharge point, without the need for any human intervention. This providential recovery of the natural environment, which for a long time seemed complex and mysterious, has been the subject of many studies aimed first of all at understanding it, evaluating it and making the best use of it.

Early studies showed that self-purification is a complex natural phenomenon occurring in aquatic environments, mainly attributable to a large number of microorganisms of different species (of both animal and plant origin), which utilize and mineralize the organic substances provided by the effluent.

Temperature influences the biodegradability of organic compounds, as it affects the biological processes of the microorganisms present in the medium, as well as the pH, salinity, etc.

Types of processes involved in self-purification [Margalef 1999].

Overall, self-purification is carried out by a series of physical, chemical and biological processes that are closely interrelated and mutually dependent.

The most characteristic physical processes in self-purification are solar radiation, sedimentation and reaeration. Sedimentation causes, by its direct action, that an important fraction of suspended matter is deposited at the bottom of the channel, a fact that generally occurs when the current velocity decreases to values below 20 cm/s, forming what is known as mud banks; its subsequent degradation is very different from that experienced by the fraction that remains in suspension.

-Chemical oxidation processes, when certain dissolved reducing substances of an inorganic nature, such as sulfites, nitrites, ferrous salts, etc., are present in the aquatic environment, consuming dissolved oxygen more rapidly than those of an organic nature.

-Biological processes, of high complexity, lead to the degradation of organic matter, whether in solid, dissolved or colloidal state. This degradation is carried out by microorganisms present in the water according to reactions that depend on the conditions of the medium (temperature, dissolved oxygen concentration, depth of the current, etc.). There are two possibilities of organic matter degradation by microorganisms:

a) When dissolved oxygen is available - **aerobic** medium - these living beings consume a certain amount of this element to oxidize and decompose organic molecules into ever simpler fragments until they reach complete mineralization (heterotrophic transformation), yielding innocuous substances such as water, carbon dioxide, nitrates, phosphates, etc., and generating their own living matter.

This **aerobic degradation** can be schematized as follows:

> organic matter + oxygen + mass of microorganisms = higher mass of microorganisms + by-product + energy

b) If the concentration of dissolved oxygen is zero or very low - **anaerobic** medium - decomposition gives rise to different products such as methane, ammonia, hydrogen sulfide, mercaptans, etc., the appearance of which involves a series of undesirable phenomena, including foul odor, corrosion and toxicity. Anaerobic degradation is carried out in two phases according to the following scheme:

organic matter + mass of microorganisms = higher mass of microorganisms + intermediate products (organic acids, alcohols, etc.) + energy + intermediate products + mass of microorganisms = higher mass of microorganisms + by-products

However, the division between aerobic and anaerobic processes cannot be as strict as we have outlined, since there are a large number of bacteria that live indistinctly in one or the other medium, and even some typically aerobic and anaerobic microorganisms in certain circumstances can adapt to life in the opposite medium.

Understanding these two forms of degradation of organic matter as a first step to cover in the life cycle of any environment, it is necessary to know how to return to new inanimate organic matter from the products obtained by both heterotrophic transformation and that which takes place in an anaerobic environment. Thus, certain bacteria and chlorophyll algae consume the mineral substances obtained as by-products of aerobic degradation to synthesize their own living matter, while releasing oxygen. These organisms will serve as food for protozoa (Flagellates, Infusoria) and metazoa (Crustacea and Molluscs). In a next step, these small animals can become prey for higher organisms, even fish, if the medium contains them. Finally, when they die, their corpses are decomposed by bacterial action and the organic matter is mineralized again to close the cycle.

For all of the above, it is convenient to insist that the self-purification of a stream does not only consist of the destruction of inanimate organic matter until its mineralization, but that this is only an intermediate step that allows the generation of new living matter.

3.2 Zones in a self-purifying stream [Nebel and Wright 1999].

From the point at which a watercourse receives an important discharge loaded mainly with organic matter, until, downstream of it, it recovers the initial conditions of purity thanks to self-purification, four zones of varying degrees of pollution can be distinguished. The extent and definition of these zones will depend mainly on the flow rates of the stream and the discharge, its oxygen content, and the amount of organic matter present.

According to the now classic system of "Saprobia", the following zones are distinguished according to the predominance of one species or another: Polysaprobia, Mesosaprobia, Mesosaprobia and Oligosaprobia. https://riopesqueria.wordpress.com/2014/05/01/los-organismos-indican-la-calidad-del-agua-streblekrauter/]

Saprobiety is a state of water quality, with respect to the content of degradable organic matter that is reflected in the species composition of the community. It is the biological expression of BOD.

a) Polysaprobic Zone: It begins at the point of discharge of used water, being a zone of degradation and active decomposition.

-Appearance: characterized by visible signs of contamination, as the concentration of dissolved oxygen decreases progressively and may even reach zero. The waters have a dirty appearance with suspended solids, turbidity, etc. being unsuitable for the development of higher life, whose forms are gradually replaced by lower ones.

-Vigor: When the dissolved oxygen concentration drops below 45 percent of saturation, the fish die from asphyxiation. Metazoans are scarce, but some rotifers and larvae of various insects (genera Eristalis and Psychoda) are found. The number of bacteria is very high (1-10 million/ml), being frequent to find filamentous bacteria such as: *Sphaerotilus natans, Leptomitus lacteus, Beggiatoa alba*, etc., which form long copious filaments sometimes attached to the walls of the channel, to the bottom materials, or to any other object, especially to the stems and stones of the orillas. In this zone the waters contain organic substances such as carbohydrates, amino acids, etc., from the partial degradation of organic matter, especially if it is of urban origin. Free carbon monoxide and SH are also found, coming from the biological decomposition of proteins or the reduction of sulfates.

b) Mesosaprobia Zone...:

-Aspect: In this zone the recovery of the water current begins. The sludge deposited on the bottom is not blackish as in the polysaprobic zone, because the decomposition of organic matter is preferably aerobic and large amounts of hydrogen sulfide are not produced. Their color is usually green due to the presence of cyanophycean algae, and diverse populations such as insect larvae, mollusks and worms (annelids, polychaetes, tubifex, etc.) develop in these sediments.

Vigor: The characteristics are very similar to those of diluted sewage water; oxidation phenomena of organic matter continue to occur and the dissolved oxygen content gradually increases. The number of bacteria - ranging from 105 to 106 per ml - decreases compared to the previous zone, while the number of protozoa, rotifers and crustaceans increases progressively. There may be some fish species that tolerate wide ranges of oxygen concentration (Cyprinids, etc.). The most characteristic organisms in this zone are, among others, Cyanophyceae (*Oscillatoria tenuis*, Diptera (Chironomidae larvae, etc., also abundant Fusarium fungi). Another peculiar characteristic is the great variation of the dissolved oxygen content that takes place during the day. With the presence of sunlight the various green organisms that inhabit this area are able to perform the chlorophyll function, releasing oxygen in the process and consequently increasing its concentration in the medium. In the absence of light, photosynthesis ceases and, as the production of oxygen is obvious, the demand for this increase remains high since it is necessary to oxidize the large amount of organic matter still present and to satisfy the respiratory requirements of the aquatic flora and fauna. Such a demand can even cancel out the dissolved oxygen content.

c) Mesosaprobia Zone

Appearance: the recovery of water currents is in progress, the decomposition of organic matter is preferably aerobic, the water is becoming clean.

Vigor:-It is characterized by a marked mineralization being very advanced the recovery of the river. The number of bacteria decreases to values of 10° to 105 per ml and nitrifying bacteria appear. The presence of carbonates and nitrates gives rise to the development of some algae, including, apart from those already mentioned, Chlorophyceae and Diatoms. Due to the activity of these algae, a high concentration of dissolved oxygen is reached. In addition to this microflora, a great variety of microfauna also develops, the most significant of which are small crustaceans, bivalve mollusks and insect larvae. The presence of a greater number of fish species is indicative of the degree of recovery achieved.

d) Oligosaprobic Zone

-Appearance: In this area the contamination has disappeared and the river recovers the appearance and characteristics of clean water that it may have had previously.

-Vigor. Here the mineralization of the organic matter that is naturally present in the water is completed, and which comes mainly from the metabolic activities of the fauna and flora as well as from the decomposition of dead species. There are few bacteria (one hundred to one thousand per ml) and the concentration of dissolved oxygen is close to saturation. The plant and animal species are very abundant and varied and at the same time very sensitive to excess organic matter, indicating by their presence a good self-purification. Among them we have Chlorophyceae, certain mosses (Fontinalis, Planaria, Gammarus crustaceans, Ancylusl mollusks), as well as a large number of larval arthropods that serve as food for fish.

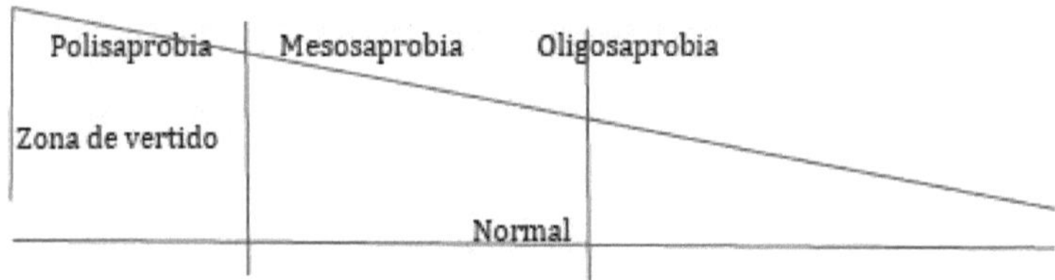

The amplitude depends on the flow rate

Figure 4 Areas with different degrees of contamination

3.3 Role of oxygen in self-purification [Odu 1971].

As a direct consequence of the above, and in a general way, it can be said that oxygen is the key element of self-purification, to such an extent that a quantitative evaluation of the content of this element in a watercourse is synonymous with a complete description of the evolution of its self-purifying process.

The oxygen content at a given time is established by the balance between those processes that involve an oxygen supply (re-aeration and photosynthesis) and those that cause a decrease in oxygen (biodegradation and respiration).

This balance can be expressed by:

O = A+F-Q-B

Being

- O= rate of change of dissolved oxygen content.
- A= oxygen transfer rate across the air-water interfacial surface.
- F= rate of oxygen production by photosynthesis.
- Q = rate of oxygen consumption by chemical action.
- B= rate of oxygen consumption by biochemical processes.

This consumption rate can be considered as the sum of the rates of in-water and bottom sludge biodegradation and respiration of living organisms. The unit for all parameters can be g O/m^3 . h.

If at any time the rate of consumption is greater than the rate of supply and production, life in water would be impossible for living organisms, except for those capable of developing in anaerobic conditions. Fortunately, photosynthesis of aquatic plant matter provides significant amounts of oxygen, and on the other hand, as the concentration of that element moves further away from its saturation value, the water is oxygenated by re-aeration from the atmosphere at a faster rate, since the driving force of the phenomenon is precisely the difference between the oxygen concentrations in the water at each instant and that corresponding to saturation.

-Factors affecting dissolved oxygen concentration

Aquatic systems are highly sensitive to all those phenomena that imply a decrease in the amount of oxygen present in them, given the low solubility of this element in water. In addition to the unquestionable incidence that the existence of a greater proportion of biodegradable organic matter will have on the oxygen content, other factors of marked influence must be considered.

Table N°1 below shows the values of oxygen concentration in water free of dissolved salts at 1 atmosphere of pressure and different temperatures:

Table N° 1 Values of oxygen concentration in water

Temperature (°C)	**Dissolved oxygen** (mg/L)
0	14,6
5	12,8
10	11,3
15	10,1
20	9,1
25	8,3
30	7

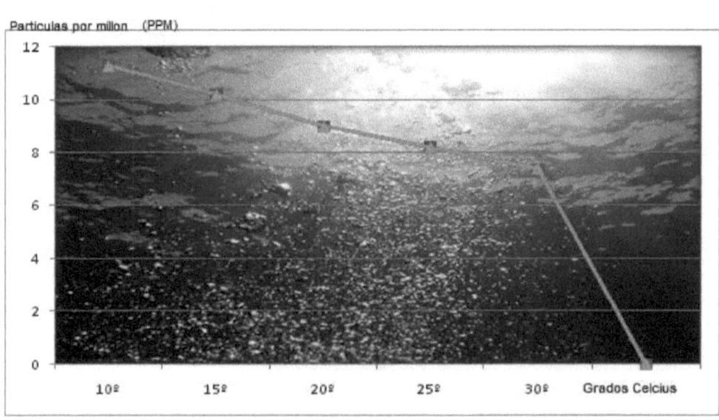

Figure 5 Oxygen Concentration (Source: https://www.tecnoaqua.es)

As can be seen, the increase in temperature has an unfavorable influence on the solubility of the gas in the liquid; but in addition, the amount of oxygen consumed by a good number of living species increases with temperature.

Another factor that negatively influences solubility is the salt content of the water.

Chemical contamination can lead to a decrease in dissolved oxygen. The existence of certain substances such as detergents, hydrocarbons, colloidal suspensions, dyes, etc., can significantly affect dissolved oxygen concentration. can significantly affect the concentration of dissolved oxygen; either by being located at the air-water interface, which is observable in the case of foams and grease films, preventing the gas absorption process in the liquid; or by preventing the entry of light into the medium and hindering the performance of the chlorophyll function by the green plants in it, an action that can also be caused by those substances that produce turbidity or provide color.

There are particularly toxic products (phenols, heavy metals, etc.) that can cause the death of some of the living species if certain concentrations - lethal doses - are reached, with the consequent increase in the organic load and decrease in the amount of oxygen produced by photosynthesis, while at the same time reducing the system's self-purification capacity by affecting the aerobic microorganisms responsible for carrying it out.

Substances that cause pH variation can alter the course of many of the processes that have to do with dissolved oxygen content.

Evolution of the oxygen content of the self-purifying stream

As described above, the oxygen content at a given point in a stream is obtained by establishing a balance between the activities that consume oxygen and those that contribute it to the water. If the longitudinal profile of dissolved oxygen in the water of a river downstream of a pollution point is represented graphically, a curve is generally obtained that has a characteristic shape called "oxygen depression curve" or "sack curve" (Figure 6).

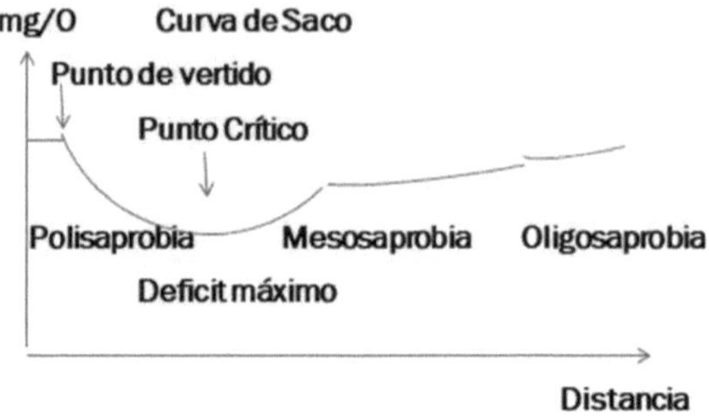

Figure 6 Oxygen depression curve or sack curve

-Critical Point -Discharge Point

The critical point where the most pronounced oxygen deficit (or the lowest concentration) is reached is located at a variable distance from the discharge point, according to the parameters just mentioned. This concentration can reach zero over a more or less long stretch, in cases of significant organic pollution, with typically anaerobic conditions then dominating, so that the clear effects of this impurification (foul smells, unpleasant aspects, etc.) are not fully felt until a certain distance downstream from the point of discharge, due to the dragging of these materials by the current and the time required for the biodegradation reactions.

Research work aimed at determining the self-purifying power of water currents in the face of polluting discharges has multiplied.

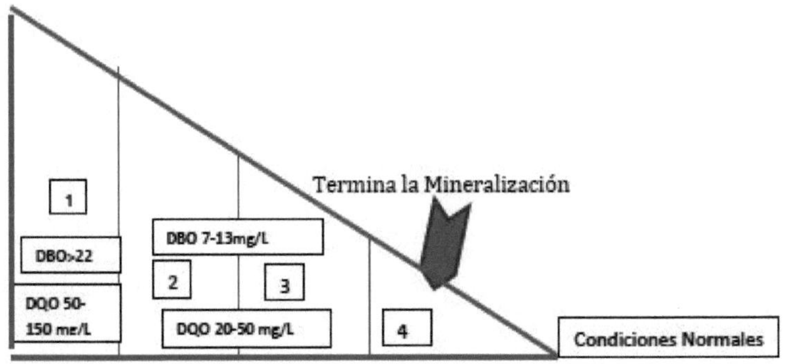

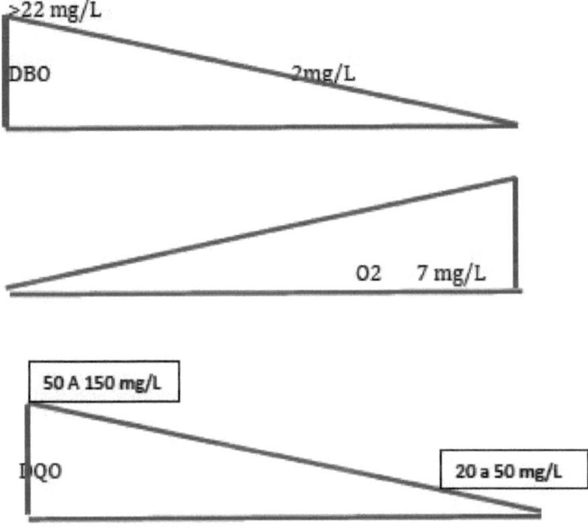

Figure 7 Evolution of a self-purifying stream

3.4 Parameters for measuring Self-Purification

Biological Oxygen Demand (BOD)

Biological oxygen demand, also called biochemical oxygen demand (BOD), is a measure of the amount of organic matter in a body of water. It is a parameter that measures the amount of matter that can be consumed or oxidized by biological means in a liquid sample, and is used to determine the degree of contamination.

It measures the amount of oxygen consumed by the action of aerobic microorganisms present in the water (degradation by microorganisms). BOD5 is normally used, which measures the oxygen consumed by microorganisms in five days. It is the most widely used organic pollution parameter and is expressed in mg O_2 /liter. A high value indicates a high presence of organic matter in the water.

Excess organic matter depletes the oxygen in the water; under these conditions the water has a cloudy, grayish appearance and odors characteristic of rotten eggs (hydrogen sulfide). This effect causes low diversity. The method measures the concentration of organic pollutants and is applicable in inland surface waters (rivers, lakes, aquifers, etc.), wastewater or any water that may contain an appreciable amount of organic matter.

Drinking water has a BOD_5 of 0.75 to 1.5 ppm oxygen, water is considered contaminated if the BOD_5 is greater than 5 ppm.

Chemical oxygen **demand**

This parameter is defined as the amount of oxygen required to oxidize organic matter under specific conditions of an oxidizing agent, temperature and time; it measures the amount of oxidant consumed during the oxidation process of all organic compounds present in water. It allows to determine the biodegradability conditions and the content of toxic substances, as well as the efficiency of the treatment units. Its determination also makes it possible to calculate the discharges of domestic and industrial effluents on the water quality of the receiving bodies.

Chemical Oxygen Demand (COD) is the amount of oxygen in mg/L consumed in the oxidation by chemical agents, whatever their origin, organic or mineral (ferrous iron, nitrites, ammonia, sulfides, potassium dichromate and others), of the reducing substances present in the water. A high value indicates water with many oxidizable substances, i.e. highly polluted.

BOD_5 and COD have so far been the two routine parameters for assessing oxygen consumption and organic load, although there are others that also complement the information and whose analysis is even faster: total oxygen demand (TOD) and total organic carbon (TOC).

3.5 Self-purification of Emerging Contaminants

The self-purification of emerging pollutants such as antibiotics, pesticides, drugs, hormones, among others, is a serious problem because many of them have a low biodegradability.

The low biodegradability of emerging pollutants explains the presence of persistent biologically active molecules, which are responsible for potential damages that can generate a loss of the capacity of a water ecosystem to self-purify itself of biodegradable organic matter.

3.6 Bibliography

Margalef R. (1999). Ecología Omega. Barcelona.

Nebel B. and Wright R. (1999). Environmental Science: Ecology and Sustainable Development, Mexico, Pearson Educación.
Odu E. (1971). Ecología, Mexico, Nueva Editorial Interamericana, 3rd edition.

Chapter 4

Farm-ecovigilance

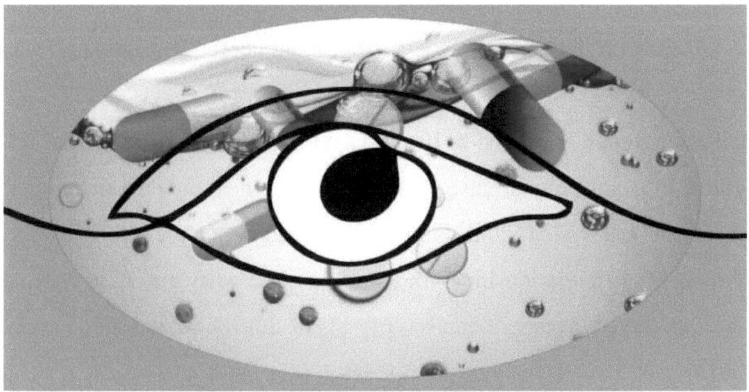

4.1 Farm-ecovigilance: A Vision with an Eco-systemic Approach

The deterioration of ecosystems has far-reaching implications for the quality of life and human health. The traditional approach to health and environmental problems neglects the fundamental fact that human health also depends on the state of ecosystems [Kummerer 2001; 2004; 2006; 2009].

The Eco-systemic approach to health [Andrade et al., 2011] approaches the issue of health from an integral perspective, where the human being is part of an eco-system and is in a continuous interaction with the environment, in a relationship with which he can modify the environment, as well as the environment can modify his health [Duncan 2001; Frangi 2000].

This interaction must be taken into account as the genesis of public health problems and for the planning of interventions. Human beings affect nature and nature affects human beings [Barragán et al, 2010].

Systems thinking and in particular the General Systems Theory (GST) [Bertalanffy 1976] is the theoretical underpinning of ecosystem approaches to human health or Ecohealth.

Systems theory understands, the presence of several interconnected elements interacting under certain limits [Mergler 2003; Mella 2017]). Several ideas included in the "umbrella of the eco-systemic approach" point out that the world in which we live can be understood as a self-organizing, holarchic and open system, which also imbues our knowledge with uncertainty [Waltner-Toews 2001].

In line with the General Systems Theory, the Ecohealth approach assumes the ecosystem as a whole. Under this principle, health is not a phenomenon isolated from other phenomena of nature and society, and is related to environmental and social aspects.

The health of eco-systems is studied [Rapport et al. 1998; Rapport et al. 2000], with a vision of prevention in human health, which is achieved with stable, healthy eco-systems, based on a culture of sustainable development [Delgado de Bravo 1996]).

The eco-systemic approach to health allows overcoming conventional schemes in the conceptions and practices of Public Health, by incorporating the environment category in the genesis of health problems [Di Pace 1992; Duran 1995] and in the intervention approaches, i.e., considering the environment as a determinant of human health, thus giving rise to the notion of environmental health (PAHO 2010).

The ecosystems and health approach has the particularity of having developed at least two approaches, one on Ecosystem Health and the other on the Ecosystem Approach to Human Health.

Ecosystem health

The approach to ecosystem health has been interpreted by some researchers as a science that integrates the natural sciences, social sciences and health sciences, concluding that it has several dimensions and attributes [De Freitas et al.]

This approach considers four dimensions:

The first dimension is biophysical, which evaluates the structures and functions of ecosystems (nutrient cycles, energy flows, and diversity of species and habitats, among others). Vigor, organization, resilience (resilience).

The socioeconomic dimension emphasizes differences in the productivity and capacity of ecosystems and the valuation of services for populations and their repercussions on economic policies.

The dimension of human health that seeks to establish a causal link between the imbalance in the state of health of ecosystems, diseases and risks to human health.

The spatio-temporal dimension considers the different responses to multiple forms of environmental stress that produce complex changes with a cumulative and/or synergistic effect that may endanger the very viability of ecosystems at the local and/or global level [De Freitas et al., 2007].

For this approach, ecosystem health is the capacity to maintain social and biological organization and the ability to achieve human objectives in a reasonable and sustainable manner.

Ecosystem health refers to the fact that there are ecosystems on earth that are unhealthy when their functions have deteriorated, especially those that are vital for sustaining the human species. This phenomenon of "unhealthiness" has been called ecosystem distress syndrome (EDS), which includes aquatic and terrestrial ecosystems. In addition to these, there is talk of different ecosystems, for example, marine ecosystems, forest ecosystems, agroecosystems, etc. [Rapport et al., 1998].

On the contrary, we can affirm that a healthy ecosystem exists when the biophysical and socio-economic functions are organized (diversity of biota and their interactions), vigorous (productivity, referring to the capacity of ecosystems to maintain the growth and reproduction of plants and animals), and resilient (capacity to buffer disturbances, capacity for recovery). The authors call these "functions" "dimensions" or "elements" that are dynamically and complexly interrelated.

Several studies on resilience of eco-social systems have focused on the capacity to absorb shocks and maintain their functions. There is also another aspect of resilience, which refers to the capacity for renewal, reorganization that is essential for sustainability processes.

In its effort to integrate the sciences, the approach assumes two perspectives that are in permanent dialogue and interaction:

-One seeks to determine how natural and artificial ecosystems function, analyzing the ways in which they function with the use of quantitative and qualitative techniques.

Another perspective is the application of transdisciplinary, evaluative strategies that assess the health of the ecosystem, considering future scenarios derived from current behavior [Rapport et al. 2000; De Freitas et al. 2007; De Freitas 2009].

Farm-ecoviglancia uses these proposals to build a theoretical and methodological framework with quantitative and qualitative techniques to detect changes in the structure and functioning of ecosystems that could be linked to urban chemical pollution produced by so-called emerging pollutants, including pharmaceuticals.

Humanity is a major force in global change and ecosystem dynamics, from local environmental forms to the biosphere as a whole. At the same time, human societies and economies worldwide are interconnected and use and impact ecosystem services.

The use of medicines in a society, an activity carried out for various purposes: scientific, economic, therapeutic or political, involves processes that are potential sources of pharmacological chemical contamination of the natural terrestrial or aquatic environment, causing ecological changes that compromise the health of natural eco-systems and therefore human health.

The eco-health approach considers human activity as the main source of environmental hazards [Novo 1996]; academic research on environmental problems does not always make this link between the world of work-environmental impact-health visible [Martin 1993].

Urban chemical contamination of the natural environment (land, water), caused by medical practice represents a danger to the health and life of human, plant and animal populations; it is a type of human or anthropogenic contamination that originates in sanitary activities, which are developed daily (Emerging Contaminants).

4.2 Pharmaco-ecovigilance: Objectives

Pharmacological science, from the moment evidence emerged of the presence of APIs in the natural environment, which were included among the emerging pollutants, assumed the objectives of eco-health and initiated research work (Farm-ecovigilance).

Among the objectives of pharmacoecovigilance are:

a) Identification, quantification and evaluation of IFA in the natural environment Development of warning systems.

a) Risk prevention: acute and chronic effects generated by contamination.

b) Incorporation of actions to optimize the effectiveness and safety of pharmacological treatments, involving all drug professionals (physicians, pharmacists, nurses, dentists) and other agents involved in the drug chain (producers, distributors, health authorities) in the safe use of drugs.

4.3 Study Areas

Farm- eco-surveillance includes studies:

Environmental -Non-Anthropocentric: studies the presence, behavior and effects of active pharmaceutical ingredients (APIs) in the natural environment, thus arriving at an environmental diagnosis of chemical contamination.

-Anthropocentric: Study of health effects on the exposed human being, public health approach.

The results of the research promote teaching actions, with a vision of prevention with central values of awareness, moderation and respect. These values represent the transition from an anthropocentric paradigm (nature as a resource and garbage dump) to a biocentric one (life in all its manifestations).

This new paradigm promotes eco-efficiency in human actions, for the achievement of an organized, healthy and sustainable eco-system.

It promotes the use of the environment in a sustainable way, without abusing it; the exploitation or contamination of the eco-system reduces its resilience, its ability to recover, which can activate a number of harmful mechanisms that endanger the health of populations.

The term **surveillance** is known as the ability to maintain attention and alertness over a prolonged period of time. Pharmacovigilance refers to the detection, supervision, monitoring, assessment and evaluation of data related to drugs in the environment and their potential hazards to human and environmental health.

In this space, pharmacological science uses to build knowledge, the convergence of methodologies from various disciplines (transdisciplinarity) being them non-experimental and experimental, in a work carried out by pharmacologists, pharmacists, chemists, biologists, ecologists, sociologists, public health officials, engineers to prevent and control pollution.

Unlike pharmacovigilance, which begins with post-marketing surveillance, eco-pharmacovigilance starts at the point of production and continues during the use of the drug in its social life, with the purpose of promoting the closing of its life cycle, in order to reduce its entry into the natural eco-system, where the drug behaves as a pollutant.

4.4 Pharmacoecovigilance: Non-Anthropocentric Research

Chemical contamination breaks the equilibrium of a natural eco-system and produces changes in its vitality; the detection of these changes can guide the search for and identification of certain contaminants.

The impact of chemical pollutants on the different levels of organization of biota through bioaccumulation and biomagnification contribute to the "environmental amplification" of the distribution of a chemical pollutant. In order to understand the behavior of these molecules, protocols are required that include in their chronograms multiple, sequential sampling in time and space, multi-species toxicity bioassays in terms of the target species used, chronic type tests and tests with mixtures of drugs, the latter to try to simulate environmental conditions and environments reasonably close to the real ones.

Sequential sampling in time and space is necessary due to the oscillations of pollutant concentrations during the course of the day, in different seasons (circadian variations), which causes the effects to be different depending on the oscillations that can be registered in the concentrations (which will be lower in rainy seasons and increased in dry seasons).

Variations at different geographical points within an eco-system express different productive activities taking place at the margins of a particular water environment.

The Environmental Assessment Criteria used are: Vigor - Productivity - Environmental Threat - Temporal and spatial variations (geographic and circadian) - Resilience (resilience, seeks to detect cumulative and synergistic effects).

The Ecohealth approach reaffirms the need to incorporate systems thinking into health and environmental research because it can lead to a better understanding of the boundaries of the pollution problem, its magnitude, and its dynamics. Ultimately, it leads to a richer and more effective research process [Charron 2012].

Since it is not possible to address them in a traditional manner due to the integrality [Botti and Giret 2008], complexity and uncertainty of the phenomena, the convergence of various disciplines is indispensable, hence the importance of transdisciplinarity.

Its approach makes it possible to address sets of problems instead of focusing on the spaces delimited by each epistemological knowledge, adopting a systemic and integrative approach to knowledge [Morin 2007; Nebel and Wright, 1999; Charron 2012].

Transdisciplinary research involves the integration of research methodologies and tools from all disciplines including non-academic perspectives and knowledge [Charron 2012].

The eco-health approach considers human activity as the main source of environmental hazards [Novo 1996]; academic research on environmental problems does not always make this link between the world of work-environmental impact-health visible [Martin 1993].

Urban chemical pollution of the natural environment (land, water), caused by medical practice represents a danger to the health and life of human, plant and animal populations; it is a type of human or anthropogenic pollution that originates in sanitary activities, which are developed daily (Emerging Contaminants).

The presence of drugs among the Emerging Contaminants that reach the environment broadens the spectrum of study of Pharmacological science in its area of surveillance, shifting its gaze from the pharmaco-epidemiological to the pharmaco-ecological space, with activities that are located at a later stage than the social life of the drug.

The ecosystem health approach is seen as a new frontier that integrates ecology, health sciences and many other fields, broadening the concept of "health-disease" from a traditional focus on the level of the individual (Clinical Medicine) and the population (Public Health) to the functions and structure of the ecosystem as a whole (Ecological Medicine) [Rapport et al. 2000].

4.5 Water quality as an indicator of eco-system status

The state of an aquatic eco-system can be known by the state of the water mass, which represents the abiotic component of that eco-system and is therefore an indicator of its health.

Water quality refers to the chemical, physical, biological and radiological characteristics of water. It is a measure of the condition of water in relation to the requirements of one or more biotic species or to any human need or purpose.

Water quality indicators can be classified in several ways:

Depending on the parameter used, they can be:

- Physical-chemical: based on physical or chemical parameters of the water such as pH, suspended solids, temperature, etc. or on a set of these parameters.
- Biological: an organism whose presence provides information on the state of health of the aquatic environment in which it develops its biological cycle. Organisms used as biological indicators of water quality are: macroinvertebrates, fish, diatoms, pathogenic organisms, etc.
- Hydromorphological: they evaluate, on the one hand, the difference between the current hydrological and geomorphological characteristics of the rivers, and on the other, the characteristics that the rivers would have in the absence of human alterations, to ensure the proper functioning of the fluvial ecosystem.

The most common standards used to assess water quality relate to ecosystem health, human contact safety, and drinking water.

4.6 Bibliography

Andrade Á., Arguedas S. and Vides R. (2011). Guía para la aplicación y monitoreo del Enfoque Ecosistémico, CEM-UICN, CI-Colombia, ELAP-U, IUCN.

CI, FCBC, UNESCO-.

Barragán H., Pascual A., Bourgeois M. and Ojeda O. (2010). Development Human Health and environmental threats. Crisis of Sustainability. Editorial of the University of La Plata.

Bertalanffy L. Von (1976). Teoría General de Los Sistemas Primera, Mexico: Fondo de Cultura Económica.

Botti V, Giret A. (2008). ANEMONA: A Multi-agent Methodology for Holonic Manufacturin Systems.

Charron D. (2012). Ecohealth: Origins and approach. In D. Charron, ed. Ecohealth Research in Practice. Innovative Applications of an Ecosystem Approach to Health. Ottawa: Springer / International Development Research Centre, pp. 1-30.

De Freitas C.M., Gomes de Oliveira S., Schütz G.E., Freitas M., Gómez Camponovo M.P. (2007). Ecosystem approaches and health in Latin America. Cadernos de Saúde Pública, 23(2), 283-296.

De Freitas C. (2009). Ecosystemic Approaches to Health: Perspectives for their adoption in Brazil and Latin American Countries First. C. Machado de Freitas, ed., Brasilia: Pan American Health Organization.

Delgado de Bravo M. (1996). Ambiente y Calidad de vida: una respuesta a los problemas de los metrópolis latinoamericanas, Buenos Aires. 55-
Dictionary of the Royal Spanish Academy (Twenty-second Edition).

Di Pace M., Feoeaovisky S., Haadoy J. and Mazzucchelli S. (1992). Urban environment in Argentina. Buenos Aires. CEAL. 202 p.

Duran R. La Argentina ambiental, Buenos Aires, 1995.

Duncan K. (2001). Ottawa Charter for Health Promotion. Public Health Educac. Health, 1(1), 19-22.

Frangi J.L. Ecology and Environment. Elementos de Política Ambiental, Honorable Chamber of Deputies, Province of Buenos Aires, 2000.

Kümmerer K. (2001). Drugs in the environment: emission of drugs, diagnostic aids and disinfectants into wastewater by hospitals in relation to other sources da review. In: Chemosphere. 45,. 957-969.

Kümmerer K. (2004). Resistance in the environment. Journal of Antimicrobial Chemotherapy 54, 311-320.

Kummerer K. and Velo, G. (2006). Ecoparmacology: A new topic of importance in Pharmacovigilance. Drug Safety 29(5), 371-373R.

Kümmerer K. (2009). The presence of pharmaceuticals in the environment due to human use present knowledge and future challenges. Journal of 7nvironmental Management 90, 2354-2366.

Martín Mateo R. El hombre una especie en peligro, Madrid, Campomanes. Libros,1993.

Mergler D. (2003). Integrating Beyond Business Process Reengineering-Towards the Holonic Enterprise.Human Health into an Ecosystem Approach to Mining. In D. Rapport et al., eds. Managing for Healthy Ecosystems. Boca Raton, Florida: Lewis Publishers, pp. 875-883.

Mella P., Gazzola P. (2017). The Holonic View organizations and Firms. Systems Research and Behavioral Science 34(3), 354-374.

Morin E., 2007. Introducción al pensamiento complejo Novena, Barcelona: Editorial Gedisa.

Nebel, B. and Wright, R. Ciencia Ambientales: Ecología y Desarrollo Sustentable, Mexico, Pearson Educación, 1999.

Novo, M. Environmental education. Ethical, conceptual and methodological bases. Madrid. Edu Universitas(1996)

PAHO, 2010. Environmental and Social Determinants of Health First. L. Galvao, J. Finkelman, and S. Henao, eds, Mexico City: PAHO/WHO.

WHO/PAHO. Health and the environment in sustainable development, Washington 2000.

Rapport D.J., Costanza R. and McMichael A.J. (1998). Assessing ecosystem health. Trends in ecology & evolution, 13(10), 397-402.

Rapport D., Hildén M. and Weppling K. (2000). Restoring the health of the earth's ecosystems: A new challenge for the earth sciences. Episodes, 23(1), 12-19.

Waltner-Toews D. (2001). An ecosystem approach to health and its applications to tropical and emerging diseases. Debate, Cad. Saúde Pública, 17(Supplement), pp. 7-36.

Chapter 5

Natural eco-system: Salí-Dulce Basin

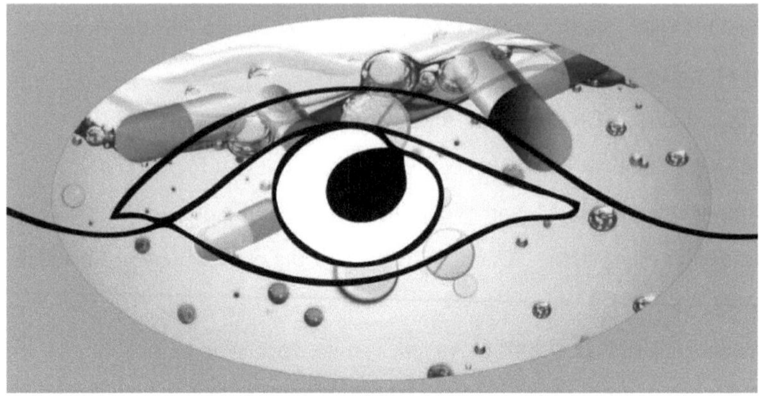

5.1 Geographic Characteristics

The Salí Dulce Basin is an area shared by the provinces of Salta, Tucumán, Santiago del Estero and Córdoba in Argentina. It occupies an area of approximately 57,320 km^2 and covers an altitude range from 200 to almost 5,500 meters above sea level. Geographically, two regions can be distinguished: the upper region in Salta and Tucumán and the lower region in Santiago del Estero and Córdoba.

In Tucumán territory, the Salí river is dammed approximately 25 km north of San Miguel de Tucumán, at the Celestino Gelsi dam (ex Cadillal), up to this point, the Salí river drains through the Tapia-Trancas basin, located in the northwest of the province of Tucumán. The second reservoir is located on the border with the province of Santiago del Estero; it is the Frontal dam, in Termas de Río Hondo.

During this second journey through the Tucuman plains, the Salí River drains the eastern slope of the Sierras del Aconquija and increases its flow considerably.

The Salí is fed by 11 rivers on its right bank and 3 on its left bank; 17 streams also drain into it. From the hydraulic point of view, all the tributaries of the Salí River are torrential in nature; they have abundant flows during the wet semester that are strongly reduced during the dry semester.

After approximately 180 km, the Salí enters the province of Santiago del Estero under the name of Dulce and flows into the province of Córdoba, in the Mar Chiquita lagoon. The Salí is a permanent river, with a predominantly north-south direction and a marked structural control. The different microclimates, the existing altitude differences, have allowed the development of plains, jungles, forests, valleys, mountains with perpetual snow, mountain rivers, a varied terrestrial and aquatic fauna. It is essential to conserve its biodiversity for the direct benefits it provides, and it is necessary to promote practices that contribute to its sustainability.

5.2 Functions of the Basin

This water system, the Salí River, provides an environmental service of fundamental importance for the agglomeration; It is the only source of permanent surface water for the entire area described, and the recipient of all the fluids used in the agglomeration. It receives, directly or indirectly, a network of drainage channels that were originally natural collectors (streams and ditches), in addition to artificial open drains, which flow into the Salí upstream (North channel) and downstream (San Cayetano and South channels) of the city of San Miguel de Tucumán.

The Salí-Dulce Watershed provides the following benefits of social interest that together are Environmental Services:

Hydrological cycles, oxygen supply, carbon dioxide uptake, climate regulation, biogeochemical regulation. It provides water for life and for the functioning of the productive system (agriculture, industry), electricity generation (dams and reservoirs). It is a source of protein through fishing, a source of wood, fruits and seeds through the pollination of flowers, a source of genes. It is also a source of recreation.

5.3 Water contamination: Waste reservoir: Pressures-Impact

The riverside sector is polluted and has a high degree of environmental degradation due to the discharge of untreated urban and industrial effluents that are discharged directly and through the network of canals.

Urban waste is generated from different sources, both by structured neighborhoods and irregular settlements without infrastructure.

Chemical pollution transforms this natural reality of environmental services; it degrades this source of resources, becoming a reservoir of substances that alter the functioning of the eco-system and harm life. [Tolcaichier 2000]

A fairly complete description of the situation in this basin was made in 1995, in the work entitled "Diagnosis of Pollution in the Salí Dulce Basin. Integral plan of action for its solution" developed by professionals of the Ministry of Science, Technology and Environment of the Republic of Cuba and the Secretariat of Natural Resources and Human Environment of Argentina, which expresses the BOD per day, shows the important industrial pollution in winter and summer, generated in winter by the sugar industry and in summer by citrus, food, yeast factories and meat processing plants. The sugar and alcohol industries generate the most pollution in the winter. Urban pollution is not considered.

Thus, one of the main sources of contamination is the contribution of industrial waste from the sugar mills, with a total of twelve distilleries, which generate approximately 1,400,000 m3 of vinasse per year, which on several occasions are discharged without prior treatment into numerous streams and rivers that finally drain - all of them - into the Salí River. This situation is further aggravated by effluents from paper mills, citrus farms, slaughterhouses, tanneries, sewage systems, and the massive use of nitrogenous and phosphorous fertilizers and pesticides, with large amounts of solid sediments and flooding [Georgieff 2012].

Pollution of the basin is a very important problem and affects the upper zone more intensely than the lower zone, which becomes the recipient of the pollution. Its receptacle is the Frontal del Río Hondo reservoir (province of Santiago del Estero), which constitutes an immense lagoon for the stabilization of organic matter.

The pollutants generated in the upper zone come from urban effluents and industrial waste. A technical-environmental analysis carried out by the Environmental Sanitation Department of SIPROSA shows which are the populations that contribute, directly or indirectly, the greatest amount of wastewater to the Salí stream, and makes it clear that San Miguel de Tucumán contributes 85.2% of the total volume of wastewater.

In 1995, the amount of solids discharged into the Salí Basin was approximately 3,600,000 tons per year, including sediments and industrial and urban effluents (sewage and solid urban waste). An important point of this study is that the effluents are mostly organic.

The poor disposal of industrial and urban waste (solid urban and sewage waste), logging and deforestation indicate that the natural system is being attacked and that there are environmental problems in the basin.

The quality of its surface waters is notably altered, the effluents discharged into the basin's rivers derive from: -Sugar industries 28% of the total effluent load, -Citriculture 13%, -Slaughterhouses 20%, -Sewage treatment plants 28%, -Bottling plants 7% and -Other activities that account for the remaining 16% of the pollutant load.

In 2013, journalist Diego Astudillo, in La Gaceta said in his article that "although biofuel production is the main pollutant, mining, landfills, sewage and agrochemicals complete a cocktail that raises doubts about its remediation. The same newspaper article explains that the main pollutant is vinasse, a waste generated in the production of ethanol using sugar cane molasses.

For many years the eleven distilleries working in Tucumán dumped this product into the river; the critical environmental situation of the Salí-Dulce basin entered strongly into the national media agenda, after the maximum environmental catastrophe in Santiago del Estero in recent years; It was in November 2011, when four tons of fish died in the Río

Hondo reservoir, generating the response of the Government and the Ombudsman's Office of that province, which promoted different judicial presentations so that the industries in Tucuman would treat their waste before discharging it into the tributary rivers of the basin. They even appealed to the Supreme Court of Justice of the Nation and presented documentation that compromises about 15 sugar mills in Tucumán [Albornoz et al, 2012].

Regarding the characteristics of the basin's liquid waste, both urban and industrial, a large amount of organic matter was detected which, upon biodegradation, consumes oxygen from the rivers for its stabilization.

Direct data on surface water quality are available at some points of the natural and artificial watercourses mentioned, such as the Salí river, El Manantial stream and North and South canals -before they flow into the Salí- and the San Cayetano canal at the intersection with Anselmo Rojas street. The controls carried out include conventional physical-chemical variables, majority ionic composition and organic contamination indicators. These can be Biochemical Oxygen Demand (BOD), Dissolved Oxygen (DO) and nutrients.

These data do not correlate with the time variable, and only some have been collected systematically as part of a Surface Water Quality Control Program. As regards wastewater treatment, the collection networks of the city of San Miguel de Tucumán are saturated in large areas. As an aggravating factor, not all of the effluent collected by these networks is treated at the San Felipe treatment plant; a large part (approximately 70%) is discharged raw, through conduits and open-air storm drains into the Salí River. Thirteen areas where this type of dumping takes place have been established [Gonzalez 2000; Puchulu 2012].

5.4 Definition of water quality variables associated with the state of a water ecosystem

Color: Impression produced by a shade of light on the visual organs. It is evaluated: with color; without color or colorless.

Smell: Sensation resulting from the perception of a stimulus by the olfactory sensory system. It is evaluated with odor; odorless or odorless.

Turbidity: Measure of the degree of transparency, due to the presence of suspended particles. It is evaluated as transparent; turbid.

Sediment: Matter that after having been in suspension in a liquid, ends up at the bottom because of its increased gravity. It is evaluated: without sediment, with sediment.

PH: A measure of acidity or alkalinity of a solution, indicating the concentration of hydrogen ions present. The pH scale varies, typically, from 0 to 14. Solutions with pH less than 7 are acidic; on the other hand, alkaline solutions have a pH greater than 7.

Temperature: Physical quantity that reflects the amount of heat in a body, an object or the environment. It is linked to the notion of cold (lower temperature) and hot (higher temperature). The unit of measurement of temperature is the degree Celsius (ºC). It corresponds to the hundredth part between the melting point of water and its boiling point on the scale that sets the value of zero degrees for melting and one hundred for boiling.

Ammonia: Chemical substance in the form of gas, with a penetrating odor. It consists of one part nitrogen and three parts hydrogen. It dissolves easily in water. It is evaluated Positive or Negative.

Nitrates-Nitrites: These are two of the nitrogen compounds that are used by plants and animals that eventually return nitrogen in gas form to the air. It is evaluated Positive or Negative.

Chloride: Chloride ion is one of the main anions in water, including sewage. In high concentrations, chloride can impart a saline taste to water. There are several methods for its determination and of these, the argentometric method is recommended for relatively clear water with Cl- concentrations of 5 mg/L or higher and where 0.15 to 10 mg of the anion is present in the titrated portion. In a neutral or slightly alkaline solution, potassium chromate can indicate the endpoint of chloride titration with silver nitrate. Quantitative precipitation of silver chloride and subsequently brick-red silver chromate occurs.

Sulfate: Sulfates are widely distributed in nature and are relatively abundant in hard water. Sulfate ion precipitates in acidic media with barium chloride forming barium sulfate crystals of uniform size. The amount of crystals is proportional to the sulfate concentration in the sample and the light absorbance of the suspension can be measured spectrophotometrically at 420 nm, the SO concentration$_4^{2-}$ being determined with respect to a calibration curve. This method allows the determination of up to 40 mg/L of sulfates. If the sample has a higher concentration, a dilution must be carried out.

Total Hardness: In practice, total hardness of water is defined as the sum of the concentrations of calcium and magnesium ions expressed as calcium carbonate in mg/L. The titrimetric method is based on the ability of the sodium salt of ethylenediaminetetraacetic acid (EDTA) to form soluble chelate complexes when added to solutions of some metal cations. When determining the Total Hardness, the pH of the solution should be around 10, for which the hardness buffer solution is added and as an indicator Eriochrome Black T, which causes a wine-red coloration. The addition of EDTA as a titrant complexes the calcium and magnesium ions and at the end point of the titration, the solution turns blue. To ensure a satisfactory end point, Mg must be present, which is introduced into the buffer. Although the sharpness of the end point increases with pH, it cannot be increased indefinitely as calcium carbonate or magnesium hydroxide would precipitate. For Calcium Hardness, sodium hydroxide is used as an alkalinizer to bring the pH to a high level in order to precipitate magnesium and to be able to determine calcium, using Murexide as an indicator, which forms with EDTA a definite violet end point. Magnesium Hardness is determined by the difference between Total Hardness and Calcium Hardness. Calcium and Magnesium are determined by calculations from Calcium and Magnesium Hardness, respectively.

Alkalinity: The alkalinity of a water is its ability to neutralize acids and is the sum of all the titratable bases. It is usually due primarily to its carbonate, bicarbonate and hydroxide content although other salts or bases also contribute to alkalinity. Its value can vary significantly with the pH of the end point. The sample is titrated with a strong mineral acid solution to pH 8.3 and 4-5.

Conductivity: Conductivity is a measure of the ability of an aqueous solution to carry an electric current. This capacity depends on the presence of dissolved ions, their absolute and relative concentrations, their mobility and valence, and the temperature and viscosity of the solution. This parameter is used to estimate the total content of ionic constituents. The physical measurement practiced in a laboratory determination is usually resistance measured in ohms. In the International System of Units the reciprocal of the ohm is the siemens (S) and conductivity is expressed in mS/m, the correspondence being 1mS/m=10 μmhos/cm. Salinity, which is dimensionless, was initially conceived as the determination of the mass of dissolved salts in a given mass of solution, but this experimental determination by desiccation presents difficulties because of the losses of some components. The only real way to determine the real or absolute salinity of a natural water is to perform a costly full chemical analysis, the accuracy of which is not always satisfactory. Thus, it was decided to determine it indirectly through different methods, among them, conductivity. This has the highest precision but responds only to ionic solutes.

Sodium: indicates salinity-Assesses Positive or Negative

Potassium**:** indicates salinity - Evaluates Positive or negative

Dissolved oxygen: Dissolved oxygen (DO) is the amount of gaseous oxygen that is dissolved in water. It is measured in mgO /L.$_2$

Chemical Oxygen Demand$_2$: Chemical Oxygen Demand (COD) is a chemical parameter, which represents a measure of all organic and inorganic matter present in solution and/or suspended that can be chemically oxidized, by the action of oxidizing agents, under acidic conditions and is measured as milligrams of "oxygen" equivalent to the dissolved and/or suspended organic fraction per liter of solution (wastewater). COD can be related empirically to BOD, organic carbon or organic matter.

Biochemical Oxygen Demand$_2$: It is one of the most widely used parameters; it is a measure of the amount of oxygen used by microbial populations in the water in response to the introduction of degradable organic material. It is measured in mg O_2 / L.

5.5 Bibliography

Georgieff SM (2012). The causes of overflows and floods in southeasternTucumán. Meeting of the Social Participation Commission of the Salí Dulce Interjurisdictional Basin Committee.June 27, 2012.

Gonzalez JA (2000), "Diagnosis of the contamination of the Salì river basin", Integral Action Plan for its solution. Cuadernos de Medio Ambiente. Superior Government of the Province of Tucumán.

Puchulu ME (2012). Diagnosis and current status of soil salinization in southeastern Tucumán. Meeting of the Salì-Dulce Basin Committee. 27 June 2012.

Albornoz M., Bollero M., Bosio M. Water and Environment. Problemática de la Cuenca Salí Dulce. Editorial UNSTA. 2012.

Tolcachier A.J. Water Pollution. Virtual Book Intramed, Roemmers, s/f 2000.

Chapter 6

Hypothesis

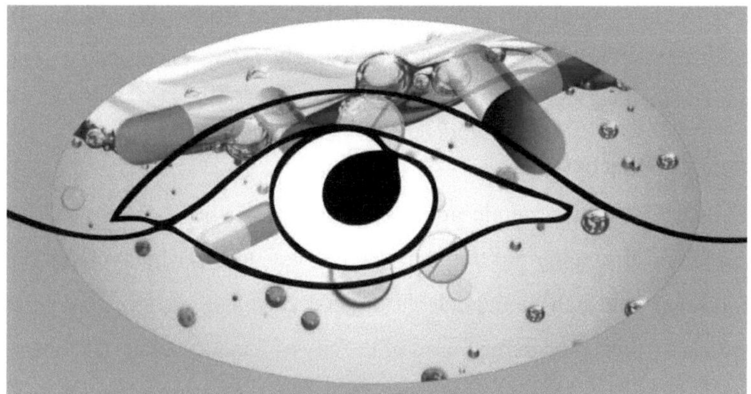

Hypothesis

The systemic approach to the problem of environmental water pollution is a useful methodology to detect changes in an eco-system. It is oriented towards the search for emerging pollutants, specifically drugs in freshwater courses, with transversal study areas that reach the Pharmacological science.

General Objective

To detect, with a systemic approach, changes in the state of a water ecosystem belonging to the Salí Dulce watershed, which could be associated with non-biodegradable organic chemical agents (Emerging Pollutants) contained in the drains of the city of San Miguel de Tucumán.

Specific Objectives

1-Delimit a water ecosystem of 100 km, belonging to the Salí-Dulce watershed and locate in it, three sub-ecosystems identified as pre-urban P1, urban P2 and post-urban P3, with different exposure to urban drainage.
2-Detect geo-temporal variations in the state of the pre-urban P1, urban P2 and post-urban P3 sub-cosystems.
3-To know the state of the water sub-ecosystem P2, which receives drainage from the city of San Miguel de Tucumán in winter and summer.
4-Analyze the variations of the self-purifying capacity of the delimited ecosystem, related to non-biodegradable organic matter.

Purpose

Contribute to the conservation of the Salí Dulce natural eco-system, a source of water and natural resources in several provinces: Salta, Tucumán, Santiago del Estero and Córdoba. The health and life of numerous populations of Northern Argentina depend on this natural eco-system.

Chapter 7

Materials and Methods

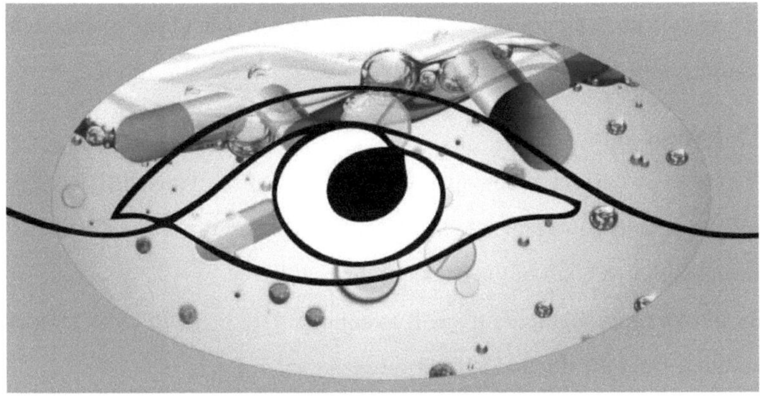

7.1 Materials and Methods

7.1.1 Type of study

Pharmacoecovigilance study; cross-sectional conducted in winter stages years 2017/2018 and summer stages 2018/2019, observational with the use of analytical techniques to determine physicochemical parameters, complemented with infrared spectroscopy and atomic absorption.

7.1.2 Study area

A system is designed, contained in the Salí Dulce Watershed System, which presents an organizational structure made up of three subsystems, located along 100 km of the banks of the Salí River.

By means of cartographic lines, it is delimited, in order to collect water samples, from the three identified subsystems.

Four campaigns were conducted, two in summer and two in winter, to monitor the water quality of the Salí Dulce Basin in three sectors of its open-air riverbed (Table 2).

Table 2 Description of sampling dates

Campaign	Date	Abbreviation
1	July 24, 2017	Jul 17
2	February 16, 2018	Feb 18
3	July 24, 2018	Jul 18
4	February 16, 2019	Feb 19

7.1.3 Sampling

A visual tour of the accessible areas of the basin was conducted. This made it possible to select the most representative sampling sites for this study. Twelve water samples were taken from the ecosystem under study, collected in winter and summer.

7.1.4 Sample collection

Sample containers:

A submerged collection bottle was used, always at the same depth. The cleaning of the container followed a pre-established protocol. The volume of water sample to be collected depended on laboratory requirements, according to the parameters to be analyzed.

Sample **preservation**

Samples for the determination of physicochemical parameters should take a simple precaution: fill the bottles completely and cap them in such a way that there is no air above the sample. This limits the interaction with the gas phase and agitation during transport, avoiding changes in the CO content$_2$ and, consequently, variations in pH. Existing methods for preservation with maximum time are limited to pH control, addition of chemicals and refrigeration.

7.1.5 Water Quality Parameters in a Water Ecosystem

Organoleptic characteristics, Physical-chemical parameters, Dissolved Oxygen, Biological Oxygen Demand, Chemical Oxygen Demand, Heavy Metals, Persistent Organic Molecules

Techniques

Temperature: A Celsius (centigrade) thermometer with a mercury column was used. The temperature was measured in situ, by direct introduction of the thermometer into the collected water.

pH: Modern pH meters (pH meters) have an electronic mechanism that automatically compensates the measurement with respect to temperature, with recording of the actual pH value at the measurement temperature. The procedure to measure this parameter is to introduce the sensor into the body of water; if this is not possible (as for deep water), the sample can be collected with one of the sampling bottles, then transferred to a completely filled polyethylene bottle (250 - 500 ml), capped and stored in the dark and at low temperature until the time of reading.

Ammonia: the indophenol blue method was used. The ammonium ion present in water reacts in an alkaline citrate medium with sodium hypochlorite. It forms monochloroamine, which in the presence of phenol and sodium nitroprusside, which acts as a catalyst, forms indophenol blue.

Nitrites: In principle nitrite NO2 - is determined by formation of a red azo compound produced at pH 2 - 2.5, coupling diazotized sulfanilamide with N-(1-naphthyl) ethylenediamine dichloride (NED dichloride). The absorbance of the solution is measured at 543 nm for subsequent quantification.

Nitrates: The main methods for evaluating nitrate ions (mg/L), in water are based on: (a) reduction to nitrite ions, and subsequent evaluation of these by colorimetric methods. (b) colorimetric reaction as a result of the oxidizing properties of sulfuric acid. (c) polarographic determination; and (d) ultraviolet spectrometry.

Chloride is one of the main anions in water, including sewage. In high concentrations, chloride can impart a saline taste to water. There are several methods for its determination. Of these, the argentometric method is recommended for relatively clear water with Cl^- concentrations of 5 mg/L or higher, with 0.15 to 10 mg of the anion present in the portion tested. In a neutral or slightly alkaline solution, potassium chromate can indicate the endpoint of chloride titration with silver nitrate. Quantitative precipitation of silver chloride and subsequently of brick-red silver chromate occurs.

Sulfates: The basis for the turbidimetric determination of sulfates (Official Method) is the reaction between the SO4 anion^{2-} and the Ba cation^{2+} to form an insoluble product. In a suspension of gum arabic it remains in solution long enough for turbidimetric analysis by spectrophotometric measurement at 425 nm.

Total hardness: method of determination is by titration with ethylenediaminetetraacetic acid (EDTA) in the presence of a buffer creating a pH of the medium between 10.0 and 10.1. The EDTA titer is previously standardized with calcium standard solution. The calcium and magnesium ions form stable complexes with ethylenediaminetetra-disodium acetate, the end point of the titration being detected by a pink to blue shift of the indicator Eriochrome-T Black. Results are expressed as mg$CaCO_3$ **/L.**

Alkalinity: method of determination by titration with standard hydrochloric acid solution of known titer validated against sodium carbonate solution. Bromocresol green indicator is used to detect the end point, until the color changes from blue to yellow. The results are expressed as mg $CaCO_3$ /L. Since the alkalinity of surface water is generally determined by the content of carbonates, bicarbonates and hydroxides, it is taken as an indicator of these ionic species (Beltran 2011).

OD: The determination of dissolved oxygen by electrometric methods offers several advantages: speed, portable instrument, continuous monitoring with signal recording equipment and less interference than chemical methods.

BOD: The BOD test is an experimental, bioassay-type procedure that measures the oxygen required by organisms in their metabolic processes that consume organic matter present in wastewater or natural waters. Standard test conditions include incubation in the dark at 20°C for 5 days. Standard test conditions include incubation in the dark at 20°C for a specified time, usually five days. Natural conditions of temperature, biological population, water movement, sunlight and oxygen concentration cannot be reproduced in the laboratory. The results obtained must take into account the above factors for proper interpretation.

Wastewater samples, or a suitable dilution thereof, are incubated for five days at 20°C in the dark. The decrease in dissolved oxygen (DO) concentration, measured by the Winkler method or a modification thereof, during the incubation period produces a BOD measurement .5

There are numerous factors that affect the BOD test$_5$, including soluble organic matter, suspended organic matter, settleable solids, floatable solids, presence of iron in oxidized or reduced form, presence of sulfur compounds, and non-homogenized (mixed) water. At present there is no methodology to correct or adjust for the effects of these factors.

CALCULUS
When the dilution water has not been inoculated: BOD_5 , mg/L = (D1-D2)/P

where:

D_1 = OD of the diluted sample immediately after preparation, mg/L,

D_2 = OD of the diluted sample after 5 d of incubation at 20°C, mg/L,

P = decimal volume fraction of the sample used.

Table 3 Water Quality according to BOD content

BOD_5 (mg/L)	Quality
50-120	Heavily polluted
30-49	Contaminated
6-29	Acceptable
'6	Good Quality

Biochemical Oxygen Demand (BOD_5) It is inversely proportional to the oxygen content (low oxygen content/high BOD content).5

COD: the oxidizable organic and inorganic substances present in the sample are oxidized by closed reflux in acid solution ($H_2 SO_4$) with excess potassium dichromate ($K_2 Cr O_{27}$) in the presence of silver sulfate ($Ag_2 SO_4$), which acts as a catalytic agent, and mercuric sulfate ($HgSO_4$) added to avoid interference from chlorides. After digestion, the remaining $K_2 Cr2O_7$ is titrated with ammoniacal ferrous sulfate to determine the consumed. Organic matter is calculated in terms of equivalent oxygen. [Baird, E. and Rice E., 2015).

Complementary analytical techniques

Infrared Spectroscopy

The region of the electromagnetic spectrum known as the infrared (IR) ranges from the red end of the visible spectrum (~0.75 μm) to the microwave region (300 to 400 μm). The fundamental IR comprises the area from 2.5 μm to 16 μm and is very useful for the study of structures. Several organic functional groups show characteristic absorptions in this region, which are used for diagnostics. The energy, between 14.3 and 1.8 kcal, is associated with fundamental IR radiation because it is insufficient to promote to an excited state. The magnitude of the energy involved in the fundamental IR is only sufficient to cause vibrational changes or deformation of chemical bonds. However, not all molecular vibrations give rise to absorption of IR radiation. Electromagnetic theory establishes that there will be absorption when the variation of the dipole moment (μ), with respect to the displacement, is different from 0. Therefore, only those vibrations that produce a variation of the dipole moment will be active.

The IR spectra were obtained on a FT-Perkin Elmer 1600 Series FT-Perkin equipment of the Institute of Physical Chemistry of the Faculty of Biochemistry, Chemistry and Pharmacy directed by Dr. Aida Ben Altabef.

Atomic Absorption Spectrophotometry

Atomic absorption analysis is based on the number of electrons associated with the nucleus of each element. The normal and most stable state of an atom's orbital configuration is known as the ground state. If energy is applied to an atom, it will be absorbed and an electron promoted to a less stable state known as the excited state. From this unstable state the atom will return to its ground state, releasing light energy.

In the ground state an atom absorbs light energy at a specific wavelength to pass to the excited state. If the number of atoms in the light path increases, the amount of light absorbed also increases. By measuring the amount of light absorbed, a quantitative determination of the amount of analyte can be made. The use of special light sources and a careful selection of wavelengths make it possible to determine specific elements.

The analysis of heavy metals by atomic absorption spectrometry is carried out on filtered samples to determine soluble metals, or on unfiltered samples subjected to acid digestion to determine total metals. This method, which is applied to analyze surface and waste water samples, is used to determine Cadmium, Chromium, Copper, Lead, Nickel and Zinc. These analyses were carried out at the LABTRA Trace Chemical Analysis Laboratory of the National University of Tucumán, directed by Dr. Adriana Sales.

Statistical analysis

Results are expressed as mean ± SEM. Differences in mean values were evaluated by analysis of variance (ANOVA). Tukey's test was used for all pairwise multiple group comparisons. In all statistical analyses, values of $P > 0.05$ were considered nonsignificant.

7.2 RESULTS

The results, corresponding to the parameters studied and measured in this work, are expressed with spatio-temporal distribution in the watercourse. In addition, infrared spectroscopy and atomic absorption analyses were performed to detect organic pollutants and trace metals, thus providing a better interpretation of the results obtained.

7.2.1 - Peri-urban sub-ecosystem, 100 km long, in the Salí Dulce Basin

The delimited eco-system belongs to the Salí Dulce hydrographic basin (Figure 2), over a distance of 100 km. Three sub-ecosystems are located in it: a) El Timbó-Departamento de Burruyacú- Prov. de Tucumán (P1: Pre-urban); b) El Bracho (P2: Urban) and c) Termas de Rio Hondo, Prov. de Santiago del Estero (P3: Post-urban) with different exposure to urban drainage in which Emerging Contaminants are mobilized.

.

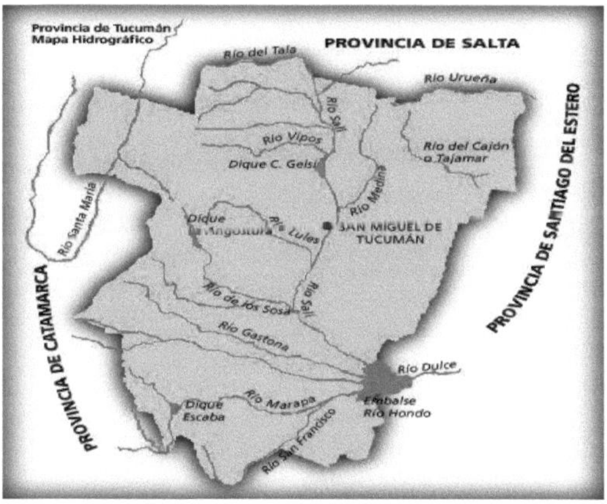

Figure 8 --Location of the Salí Dulce Watershed

The sub-ecosystem called P1 (pre-urban) corresponds to a rural area, located after the Celestino Gelsi reservoir and before reaching the urban area (San Miguel de Tucumán). It shows low urbanization and high agricultural development, so it is a site of interest for evaluating the quality of the basin, since it could receive polluting agrochemicals through surface runoff. The presence of ammonium and phosphates, the latter associated with the use of fertilizers in the productive sector, would be evidence of what was postulated in the previous paragraph.

Sample site P2 (urban). It is a highly urbanized area, with high vehicular traffic, which also houses some industries. The presence of settlements on the banks of the stream suggests potential contamination, mainly direct discharges of human waste associated with the absence of a sewage service network. Area of greatest potential contamination.

Finally, site P3, post-urban, is a rural area 70 km from the urban area, before the stream enters the Termas de Rio Hondo Dam. It is of interest to know the water quality at this site because it influences the lower section, which flows into the Termas de Rio Hondo Dam.

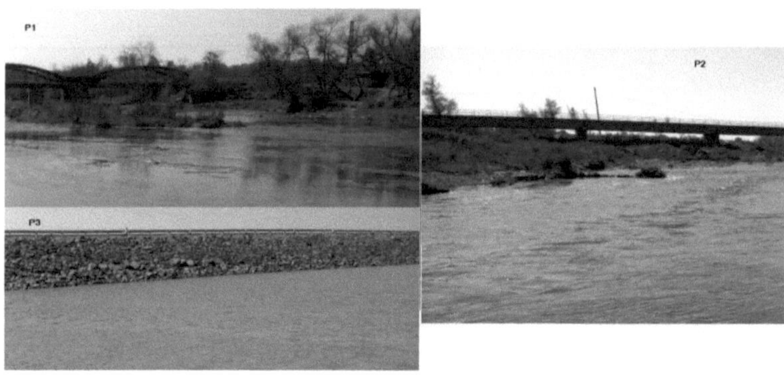

Figure 9 Sampling sites

Table 4 Geographical location of sampling sites

Geographical coordinates				
Site	Location	Latitude	Length	H
P1	El Timbo	26°43' 08 "S	65°09' 45 "O	487 masl
P2	El Bracho	26°58 20 "S	65°13' 52 "O	382 masl
P3	Termas de Río Hondo Reservoir	27°31'16 "S	64°52'56 "O	251 masl

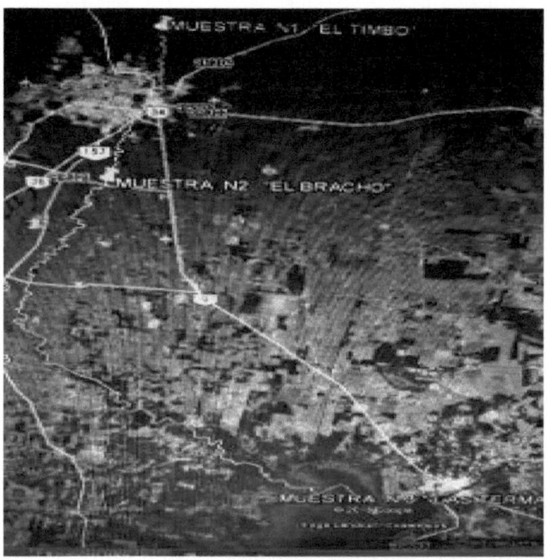

Figure 10 Geographic location of the three sampling sites (Source: own elaboration).

7.2.2 Condition and seasonal variations of the watershed sub-ecosystem designed in this study

7.2.2.1 Organoleptic characteristics

Table 5 shows marked seasonal variations in the organoleptic characteristics of the water, winter modifications in color, odor, and turbidity of the samples taken.

Table 5 Organoleptic characteristics

Time of year	Parameters	Values Normal	Item 1	Item 2	Item 3
INVERNAL	Temperature	NR	17,0 ± 1,0	12,0 ± 1,0	15,0 ± 1,0
	Color	No color	Colorless	Not	Colorless
	Odor	Odorless	Inodora	Particular	Inodora
	Turbidity	1-8 NTU	2,5±0,1	20,0±0,1	15,0±0,1
	Sediment	Scarce	No	Scarce sediments	No sediment
ESTIVAL	Temperature	NR	24,5 ± 1,0	22,0 ± 1,0	25,3 ± 1,0
	Color	No color	Colorless	Colorless	Colorless
	Odor	Odorless	Inodora	Inodora	Inodora
	Turbidity	1-8 NTU	6,0 ± 0,1	8,0 ± 0,1	3,0 ± 0,1
	Sediment	Scarce	Scarce	Scarce	No sediment

N.R.= Not Referenced

There are seasonal variations in the organoleptic characteristics of the water. Signs of deterioration in water quality can be observed in P2, mainly in the winter stage. The water temperature is linked to the irradiation received, being the temperatures measured both in the summer and winter stage compatible with aquatic life. Colored substances, suspended matter, clay, silt, organic colloids, plankton and microscopic organisms modify the color and determine the turbidity of the water. In the winter stage, water samples in P2 are not colorless: indicating the presence of suspended matter. According to WHO (World Health Organization), the turbidity of water for human consumption should never exceed 5NTU, and should ideally be below 1NTU UNF/NTU. Turbidity is measured in Nephelometric Turbidity Units In the winter stage turbidity is 12NUT and in the summer stage 8NTU for P2, considered the sub-ecosystem with the most altered organoleptic characteristics.

7.2.2.2 Physical-chemical parameters

The chemical components also show seasonal variation as shown in Table 6.

Table 6 Physical and Chemical Parameters

Season of the year	Parameters	Item 1	Item 2	Item 3
Winter	**Nitrites [mg/L]**	ND	ND	ND
	Nitrates [mg/L]	ND	15,53 ± 2,4	ND
	Chlorides [[mg/L]]	0.525 ± 0.2 (Vn 0.5-2)	0,925 ± 0,1	0,600 ± 0,1
	Sulfate [mg/L]	110.0 ± 15.0 (Vn	105,0 ± 21,0	115,0 ± 12,0
	Total Hardness [mg	19.85 ± 1.9 (Vn 10-15)	25,35 ± 2,7	13,65 ± 3,4
	Alkalinity [mg $CaCO_3$	140,5 ± 33,1	178,26 ± 28,3	174,00 ± 18,0
	Ammonium [mg/L].	3,5 ± 0,2	4,1 ± 0,5	2,1 ± 0,3
	Calcium [mg/L].	58,0 ± 2,9	90,0 ± 2,0	40,0 ± 3,0
	Magnesium [mg/L].	7,0 ± 2,0	15,0 ± 2,0	5,0 ± 2,0
	Sodium [mg/L]	106,0 ± 15,0	136,0 ± 10,0	50,0 ± 9,3
	Potassium [mg/L].	9,0 ± 1,0	11,2 ± 1,0	6,2 ± 1,0
	Electrical conductivity (EC)	886 ± 15,0	1082 ± 19,0	905 ± 11,0
	Total Dissolved Solids (TDS) $[mg.L]^{-1}$	618,0 ± 12,0	692,0 ± 20,0	587 ± 16,0
	pH	7,50	8,50	8,61
Estival	**Nitrites [mg/L]**	ND	ND	ND
	Nitrates [mg/L]	4,9 ± 2,0	11,6 ± 3,6	ND
	Chlorides [mg/L]	1,40 ± 0,1	0,60 ± 0,1	0,85 ± 0,1
	Sulfate [mg/L]	92,0 ± 10,0	100,0 ± 29,0	89,0 ± 15,0
	Total Hardness [mg	13,6 ± 2,4	16,0 ± 2,3	11,10 ± 1,8
	Alkalinity [mg $CaCO_3$	110,5 ± 25,6	132,5 ± 19.7	110,0 ± 22,4
	Ammonium [mg/L].	2,1 ± 0,3	2,8 ± 0,1	1,9 ± 0,5
	Calcium [mg/L].	40,0 ± 2,5	75,0 ± 1,5	25,0 ± 1,9
	Magnesium [mg/L].	7,0 ± 0,9	11,0 ± 0,9	4,0 ± 0,9
	Sodium [mg/L]	99,0 ± 5,6	114,0 ± 5,0	87,0 ± 7,0
	Potassium [mg/L].	8,7 ± 1,0	9,1 ± 1,0	7,9 ± 1,0
	Electrical conductivity (EC)	1110 ± 20,0	1291 ± 15,0	998 ± 12,0

	Total dissolved solids (TDS) [mg.L]-1	345,0 ± 17,0	489,0 ± 20,0	399,0 ± 22,0
	pH	6,10	6,00	7,25

ND: not detected

In the winter stage, an increase in salt concentration is observed. Higher pH values were also observed in the winter season. The pH values were within the range of 6.50 to 8.61 upH. In general, all sampling sites in the winter season presented acceptable pH values. However, in the summer season, the P1 and P2 subecosystems presented slightly acidic pH, which could be due to increased decomposition as a consequence of important organic matter discharges in that sector of the basin.

Conductivity is related to the content of dissolved ions, to the concentration of total solids in solution and to the temperature of the medium (APHA, 1998). The seasonal variation of this parameter correlates directly with the seasonal variation of temperature, presenting the highest conductivity values in the season of higher temperature. Therefore, this behavior is expected according to the temperature differences between sampling campaigns, since a 2% increase in conductivity is estimated with a 1°C increase in water temperature (Barron and Ashton, 2005). The EC value is influenced by the concentration and composition of dissolved salts. The higher the EC value, the higher the salinity present. It is important to consider that all inorganic fertilizers are salts and therefore have a direct effect on the EC. The dissolved solids content is also higher in the winter stage. Ammonium, nitrite and nitrate were not detected.

7.2.2.3 Dissolved Oxygen, Biochemical Oxygen Demand and Chemical Oxygen Demand

Dissolved oxygen (DO) is one of the most important elements in aquatic ecosystems, since its presence and concentration determines the species, according to their tolerance and range of adaptation, establishing the structure and functioning. The low concentration of dissolved oxygen in water is generally an indication of high organic pollution.

As shown in Table 7, the DO concentration at P2 is 1.9±0.3 mg/L at a water temperature between 12°C and 17°C (normal value: 11.3 mg/L - 10.3 mg/L); while in summer the value detected is 104.0+-28 mg/L, whereas the expected value for a water temperature between 20 and 25°C would be 9.1 mg/L - 8.3 mg/L. The DO concentrations exceed the expected values at this critical point, where urban effluents loaded with organic waste are received.

Table 7 Dissolved oxygen, Biochemical Oxygen Demand and Chemical Oxygen Demand

Season of the year		**Item 1**	**Item 2**	**Item 3**
Winter	**DO** (mg/L)	13,5 ± 1,7	1,9 ± 0,3	22,3 ± 8,2
	BOD_5 (mg/L)	3,3 + 0,2	-------	7,7 ± 1,5
	COD (mg/L)	20,5 ± 2,9	41,8 ± 2,2	19,1 ± 1,7
Estival	**DO** (mg/L)	78,0 ± 15,0	104,0 ± 28,0	59,2 ± 12,8
	BOD_5 (mg/L)	58,2 ± 10,1	5,6 ± 1,4	43,4 ± 11,3
	COD (mg/L)	29,0 ± 3,2	37,8 ± 1,2	21,8 ± 1,9

In the winter stage, oxygen consumption by the microbiota is not detectable in the samples obtained. In the summer stage, there is hyperoxygenation of the water, with a BOD typical of water that is not very polluted. The COD expresses oxidative activity on non-biodegradable organic matter, with values lower than expected. The values of BOD_5 and COD do not correspond to a geographical point of reception of urban waste, where it is expected to find streams with significant organic pollution.

7.2.2.4 Qualitative Analysis by Infrared Spectroscopy

Qualitative water analysis by infrared spectroscopy is a rapid method to determine the presence of analytes in a contaminated water matrix [Castillo-Bertel et al 2013]. Different functional groups and types of bonds have different frequencies and absorption intensities. In Table 8 we present the diagnostic value signals and spectra corresponding to water samples P1, P2 and P3 in the winter and summer stage, respectively.

Table 8 Diagnostic value signals observed in infrared spectra

Assignment	Normal ranges (cm-1)	Remarks
O-H	4000 - 3100	Dominated mainly by a very broad band due to O-H bond stretching
-CH Csp3-H	3000-2850	Corresponds to the C-H stretch
-C=O	1800- 1500	Corresponding to esters, Amide I and Amide II
$-C-CH_3$ $C-CH_2$ with CH_2 or CH_3	1470-1450	Scissor Vibration CH_2 and CH_3 (Narrow)
$-CH_3$ $-CH(CH\ )_{32}$	1375	Deformation of C-H bond in iso-groups (medium tight)
$-C-(CH_2\ )n-C$	720-725	Chain balance of at least 4 CH groups$_2$ (average)

These results highlight the residual presence of organic molecules in the water samples evaluated.

WINTER

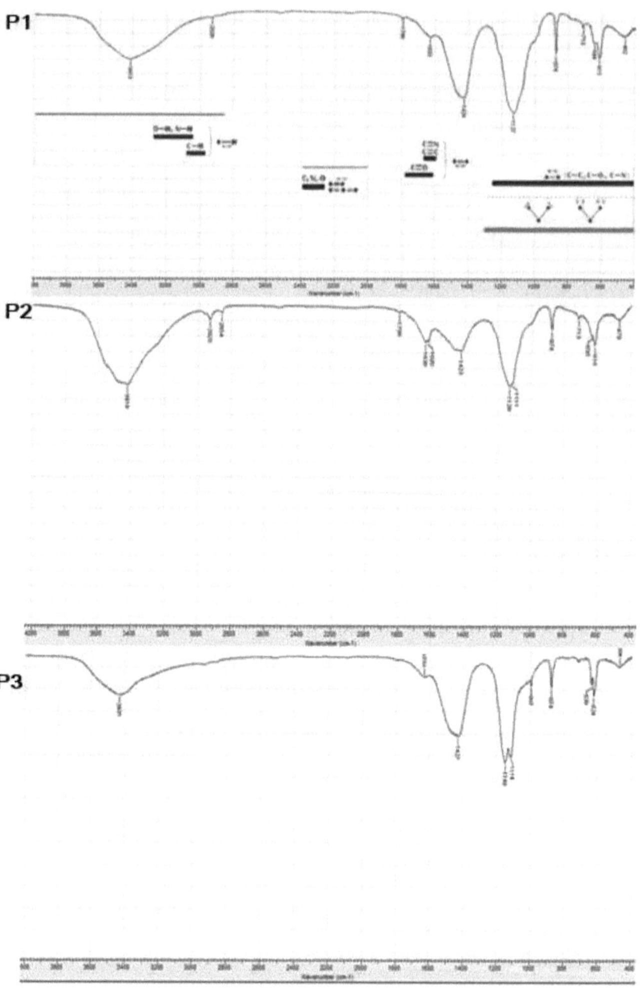

Figure 11 Infrared spectroscopy of water samples obtained from sampling points during the winter season.

SUMMER

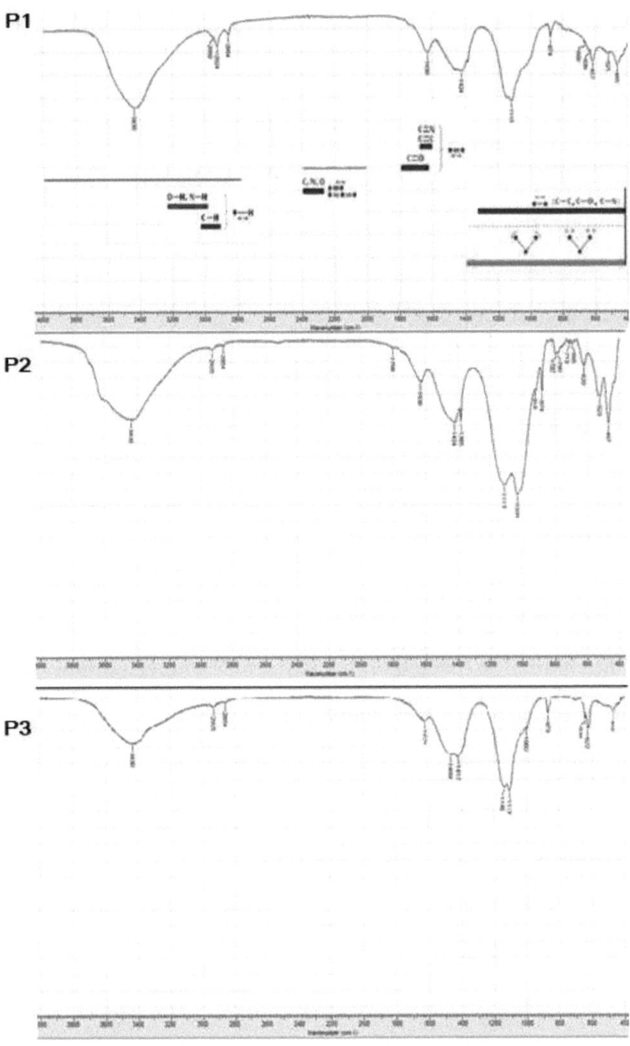

Figure 12 Infrared spectroscopy of water samples obtained at the 3 sampling points during the summer season.

7.2.2.5 **Atomic** Spectrometry Analysis

The presence of heavy metals was analyzed by atomic spectrometry in

P2, during the winter stage, considered the most altered with respect to quality characteristics.

Heavy metals are generally found as natural components of the earth's crust, in the form of minerals, salts or other compounds. They cannot be easily degraded or destroyed naturally or biologically since they do not have specific metabolic functions for living beings (Méndez et al. 2009). The results are presented in Table 9.

Table 9 Inorganic contaminants (metals)

Metals	P2 El Bracho	
Lead (U/L)	2,450 ± 0,600	(VN 0,300 U/L)
Arsenic (U/L)	ND	(VN ≤ 0.010 U/L)
Cadmium (U/L)	ND	(VN ≤ 0.005 U/L)

Atomic absorption spectrometry detected, in the case of Lead, values well above the normal expected value. Arsenic and Cadmium were not detected. They can reach a water supply system as industrial waste dumped without prior treatment. They are subsequently deposited in lakes, rivers and various aquifer systems (Duffus, 2002). In crops, the accumulation of heavy metals is the result of their uptake by irrigation with contaminated water, via roots or by deposition of airborne particles on foliage (Mor and Ceylan, 2008).

7.3 DISCUSSION

Ecological Medicine considers the state of health of natural ecosystems as determinants of human health, and for this reason evaluates the interaction of urban ecosystems with natural ecosystems. This interaction favors the chemical contamination of rivers, produced by riverside cities, an important obstacle for the sustainability of a water ecosystem and for human health. The sustainability of the natural ecosystem is compromised when receiving urban drainage that transports biologically active chemical molecules, mostly of synthetic origin known as Emerging Contaminants [Barceló and López 207]. Among them are active pharmaceutical ingredients [API]. To detect the presence of molecules of pharmaceutical origin in an aquatic environment contaminated with organic and inorganic matter, pharmacovigilance uses a theoretical and methodological framework different from that used by pharmacological science in previous study stages. The applied study process, to identify pharmacological chemical residues (IFA) [Becerril 2009], in surface water of a river, requires transversal thoughts and actions, which unite Pharmacological science with Ecology. It is a Systems Approach that draws on General Systems Theory. The General Systems Theory (GST) allows a holistic view of the different phenomena and processes of this ecological reality of chemical contamination. It is a useful tool for understanding living systems and for predicting future processes [Bertoglio, 1993]. It makes it possible to define and apply preventive measures to minimize or avoid alterations in the natural environment. Chemical pollution, favored by the interaction between open urban and natural ecosystems, with continuous bidirectional flow of matter and energy between them, can affect their organization and equilibrium.

According to the Dictionary of the Royal Spanish Academy, urban is that which "belongs or relates to the city". From an environmental perspective, it represents an energy-consuming and waste-producing space that eliminates pollutants derived from its endogenous metabolism. The pollutant load that enters the natural ecosystem breaks its equilibrium and activates internal self-regulation processes to recover homeostasis. This characteristic contributes to the maintenance of the system over time without losing sustainability, which is the emergent property of a system. The pollutant load or mass load represents a measure of the mass of pollutant per unit of time, discharged by a waste stream, expressed in Kg/d, T/day or Tons/year). In an urban drainage system, organic matter predominates and contains the molecules of the IFAs.

Studying the state of health of the receiving eco-system [Rapport et al. 1998; Rapport et al. 2000], makes it possible to detect modifications of the natural environment into which they enter and which can be attributed to them. The state of health of a natural ecosystem is maintained by respecting the fulfillment of internal processes that maintain life in it.

In order to determine the state of health of the natural ecosystem of the Salí Dulce watershed, a model was constructed, with a delimitation within the watershed, covering an area of 100 km, considered as a unit that contains 3 sub-ecosystems, which are at the same hierarchical level. Each sub-ecosystem has a different geographic location: P1 pre-urban, P2 urban, P3 post-urban, which defines different exposure to the drainage of the city of San Miguel de Tucumán. This systemic model is reminiscent of the structure of the Russian mamushka doll. The three identified sub-ecosystems are unidirectionally related by aquatic currents that move through the basin from P1 to P3. Vital processes take place inside the ecosystem, delimited by 100 km, and the urban system interacts with it on the outside.

The internal vital processes were analyzed in each identified subunit. Interdependence is a characteristic of their behavior; the imbalance of any one of them causes the imbalance of the whole. The "*whole is more than the sum of its parts*"; this allows predictions to be made about the state and behavior. Systems theory contains basic premises that are employed in this study: systems when open imply constant exchange with their environment. Both urban and natural systems are open and hierarchical, i.e. with levels of organization, the delimited natural one containing the subsystems indicated. The functions of each system depend on its structure. This implies that the loss of a sub-system, regardless of its hierarchical level, has consequences for adjacent systems and for the hierarchically superior system. There are two central concepts in general systems theory, homeostasis and feedback. Homeostasis is the capacity to respond to the variations that may exist in its environment, in order to maintain its internal environment constant.

However, this does not mean that the internal environment is immutable, but that it fluctuates within safe parameters for the system. In the natural eco-system under study, the P2 subunit receives the organic matter, the main incoming pollutant, and according to its nature it will or will not be degraded in this environment. The active pharmaceutical ingredients [API] chemical residues of used drugs represent mostly synthetic molecules that are not degraded in the natural environment they enter. These non-biodegradable molecules define a hazard. Their biological activity is capable of generating deleterious modifications in the natural ecosystem by impacting on different levels of the biota. Biota is understood as the set of living organisms (prokaryotes and eukaryotes) that occupy a given place. The processes that take place in the eco-system influence water quality and therefore biodiversity. Damage to the biota modifies the state of the exposed ecosystem, altering its structure and functions. Consequently, it cannot sustain life, which is known as Ecosystem Distress Syndrome. The P2 subunit in this research is the entrance door of the urban pollutant load to the delimited water system. Thus, its evaluation expresses a state of distress with compromise of its vitality and therefore sustainability. The health status of P2, compared to the health status of the other sub-units belonging to the same hierarchical level, presents a greater compromise. The geographical location with greater exposure to urban drainage allows inferring that the modifications detected at this point would be an expression of the environmental impact produced by the reception of this load. To reach this conclusion, the state of health of each of the sub-units was analyzed, which is expressed in the fulfillment of internal processes. The study of internal processes allows us to know the permanent interaction between the biotic and abiotic components, in order to favor the continuous flow of matter and energy, necessary to maintain life. The biocentric paradigm of the eco-systemic approach, focused on sustainability and biodiversity, considers water quality as the capacity to maintain life in the aquatic ecosystem. That quality depends on the concentration of dissolved oxygen in it and its variations. Local variations in dissolved oxygen express the capacity of each subunit to self-purify through internal oxidative metabolic processes. In P2, the concentration of dissolved oxygen in the water does not correspond to what is expected for a geographical point of reception of organic pollutant load, that is, low concentrations of oxygen in the water, produced by the aerobic metabolism of the microbiota (Figure 6 sac curve). In the samples of the first sampling, in the winter and summer stages, there is hyper-oxygenation in the water, which increases in the summer. In the second sample taken in the winter stage of the following year, the hyper-oxygenation is replaced by a state of severe hypoxia incompatible with life, with no detectable BOD. If oxygen is the vital element of a water ecosystem, these abnormal concentration variations in the samples obtained indicate the internal functionality. In the geographical point under study, they are modified since oxidative biodegradation, an aerobic metabolic process that generates a decrease in oxygen in the water, caused by decomposing microorganisms, is not perceived (Figure 6 sac curve). In other words, they transform organic matter into inorganic matter (mineralization process), which serves as a nutrient for the producing microorganisms and plants.

They, in turn, transform light energy into chemical energy, a whole internal life cycle of an ecosystem, which is altered when biodegradation is modified. Hyperoxygenation may result from human intervention in the sewage treatment plant, located in the vicinity of the geographical point under study, which attempts to mitigate chronic states of anoxia generating anaerobic metabolism and local putrefaction. It is a damaged ecosystem, which human intervention seeks to compensate. The P2 subunit is an unhealthy sub-ecosystem, incapable of sustaining life in all its manifestations; the oxygen concentrations found allowed us to deduce that biological self-purification is not fulfilled. Thus, the biodegradable organic load becomes a pollutant of the receiving ecosystem. The microbial population of the water samples obtained in the geographic point under study showed activity that could not be recorded in terms of BOD. As it is a receptor of urban drainage with a high organic load, BOD $values_5$ are expected to express an important oxygen consumption, characteristic of an aerobic microbial metabolism.

The BOD_5 , not detectable in the P2 samples during the winter stage, *defines suspicion of the presence of toxic substances*, with a broad-spectrum deleterious impact on the microbial population. The P2 samples in the summer stage show a microbial activity that remains depressed and the BOD $values_5$ obtained would correspond to streams not contaminated with organic matter. This situation is contrary to the point of reception of urban drainage, which confirms the compromised functional state of the microbial population. Climatic factors influence the functioning of the sub-unit (delimited ecosystem), which shows seasonal variations. During the winter, rainfall is scarce, in addition to the increased local agro-industrial activity with the disposal of agrochemical waste into the basin. The low flow favors water contamination by urban waste, which would explain the BOD $results_5$ in the samples obtained during the winter. Chemical aggression is one of the factors that can modify microbial activity. The BOD $values_5$ obtained allow us to conclude that there is an Environmental Impact or Environmental Footprint related to the urban mass load, made up of biodegradable organic matter, non-biodegradable organic matter and inorganic matter. In the samples studied, inorganic matter was detected due to the presence of Pb and other metals, which moved in a medium with pH>7. Alkalinization of the water was determined during the winter stage, typical of organic contamination; factors also indicators of damaged microbiota. According to what was analyzed, the *bioassay*, in addition to being an *indicator of contamination* by organic matter in the water, is an *indicator of the activity of the microbial population* present in the samples studied, which allows us to know the interaction between biotic/abiotic components of the ecosystem. Multi-causality, characteristic of complex thinking, is a fundamental part of the systemic approach. In contrast, positivist scientific reasoning considers multi-causality a limitation because it seeks to establish linear cause-effect relationships. The COD results, in the P2 samples, indicate the presence of non-biodegradable molecules in the environment considered and, together with inorganic matter, could be co-responsible for the biocidal effect on the microbiota. It was not possible to establish a BOD/COD ratio, useful for studying the composition of the biodegradable/non-biodegradable organic mass load. Among the non-biodegradable matter are molecules of emerging pollutants of urban origin, with potential harmful effects on the biota of the ecosystem. Biocides are added to many consumer goods to prevent the development of microorganisms [Barceló and Petrovic 2007]. They are used as disinfectants, antiseptics, herbicides, insecticides, cosmetics, antibiotics. Biocides in contact with the microbiota can induce lysis and also resistance to the substances with which they interact, determining the selective survival of resistant bacteria [Dang et al. 2007]. The scientific literature, referred to pharmaco-ecovigilance, reported the presence of biocides in urban wastewater, before entering and leaving the Sewage Treatment Plants. The damaged microbial population of these stations represents a weakness of the protective barrier of the natural environment [Lindström, A 2002].

There are chemical agents, of therapeutic use such as antibiotics, that exert biocidal actions. In the Suquía river, in Argentina, the presence of antibiotics, identified as belonging to the quinolones group, was detected [Valdez et al 2014]. This work adds evidence of the presence of antibiotics in freshwater courses in different countries of the world. These compounds remain in the water or precipitate, being deposited in the sludge of ecosystems with the potential for bioaccumulation and biomagnification. The presence of biocides in the urban drainage water of the city of San Miguel de Tucumán could explain the BOD values obtained. For this purpose, it was necessary to search for and identify this class of molecules in urban wastewater, before entering and leaving the wastewater treatment plants. The investigation included surface water and also the above-mentioned deposition sites in the basin. The search was oriented towards the antibiotics most used by the population of San Miguel de Tucumán. This objective required specifying the search points, taking into account the state of the ecosystem in which the molecules are found and the potential kinetic behavior they will have. The role of Waste Liquid Treatment Plants is fundamental to avoid the entry of emerging contaminants into the natural environment [Gil 2012; Rivera-Utrilla, 2013; Delgado 2011]. Several investigations reported on the limitations of WWTPs that rely on conventional treatments to remove contaminants. In addition, chemical pollutants can alter the biodegradation processes that are carried out in them, with detriment to the procedures used to degrade the incoming material. For this reason, the contamination of drainage water increases [Kolpin 2002; Ratola 2012)]. A characteristic of the holistic systemic vision is the possibility of detecting different problems that have an impact on the problem under study and also of understanding the relationships between the system and its context. In this case, the important role of the WWTPs in the preservation of the health of the natural environment. The environmental damage caused by the urban load depends on the volume of this load and its content, characteristics closely related to cultural aspects of the population that eliminates it and to the proper functioning of the urban wastewater treatment plants. The damage observed in the microbiota of the natural ecosystem under study allows us to deduce that the microorganisms of the wastewater treatment plant are also affected. According to the Rapport criteria applied in P2, vigor has been lost because it is structurally and functionally altered; its homeostatic mechanisms do not work. It is a polluted environment where life is not feasible, it loses the capacity to provide services with its resources and becomes a Red Point of environmental pollution, endangering the health of the surrounding populations. Based on our results, the drains of the city of San Miguel de Tucumán represent a threat to the sustainability of the sub-ecosystem in direct contact with them. This premise demands the design of strategies to preserve the health of the eco-system that contains them. The city of San Miguel de Tucumán is not supplied with water from the sub-system under study. However, it should be noted that around this contamination red spot, there are human settlements of marked precariousness, whose inhabitants use it as a source of resources while disposing of their waste to this eco-system, a situation that supports the concepts of the WHO, with the identification of poverty as the main cause of risk to human health. The unhealthy state of the sub-ecosystem studied shows the relationship of two urban-natural ecosystems, which when interacting allow the movement of chemical molecules in a bidirectional way. The state of sub-ecosystem P2 shows that the city of San Miguel de Tucumán pollutes and damages the natural environment with its waste. A sustainable city does not pollute, nor does it compromise the quality of a vital resource such as water. A sustainable city offers quality of life to its inhabitants, without putting resources at risk, as it respects the welfare of future generations and seeks social justice. One of the 17 Sustainable Development Goals of the United Nations is to make cities and communities sustainable. From this perspective, it is recognized that urban eco-systems are protagonists of complex relationships that obey physical and biological phenomena and that act transversally with sociology, anthropology, economics and history [Cronon 1992; Pickett et al, 1997]. From an environmental perspective, the urban context requires understanding the dynamics of a complex system and its relationship with cultural habits, where the human process of adaptation to the city must maintain balance with the natural ecosystem. With regard to APIs, economic and cultural interests favor the medicalization of life and with it the increased production of pharmacological waste. These cultural differences explain qualitative and quantitative changes in the amount of drug waste that a city can dispose of, moving it away from the ideals of an eco-city. The contamination that the mass load of the city of San Miguel de Tucumán produces in sub-unit P2 is ratified when comparing its health status with that of sub-unit P1, which is not exposed to this load. The differences detected correspond to organoleptic and physicochemical studies of the water samples obtained at both points, and ratify the environmental impact produced by the urban pollutant load. In P1 Pre-urban and P3 Post-urban, the dissolved oxygen concentrations are compatible with the development of life in the eco-system, but the low BOD values$_5$ evidence dysfunctionality of the microbiota on organic matter, so that the self-purification capacity of both geographical points is also compromised. The above description allows predicting that the vitality of the ecosystem delimited in 100 km is compromised; it cannot free itself from the biodegradable organic matter that acts as a pollutant, due to the deficient activity of the microbiota of the system. This state of contamination with biodegradable organic matter makes it difficult to reach the IFA molecules, so P2 is ruled out for searching for them, concentrating this activity on P3. Infrared spectroscopy emerges as a qualitative physical tool to detect the factors responsible for the damage to the microbiota, because they are the non-biodegradable and persistent organic molecules. There are precedents in the use of infrared spectroscopy in the study of river water contamination produced by herbicides [Somsen et al 1996]. This technique is used to identify IFA, which may be present in the water in the sludge or in the biota of the ecosystem and which represent the greatest danger of urban chemical pollution, for the ecosystem and for human health [Gil et al. 2012].

Infrared spectroscopy acts as a complement to previous studies, while the aforementioned provide a sectorial vision, spectroscopy gives a holistic view of the system. Thus, with the aforementioned technique, chemical groups of organic molecules that are mobilized throughout the delimited system (sub-units P1-P2 P3) are detected, being them of possible agro-industrial and urban origin. The physical-chemical studies of the ecosystem delimited in 100 km show seasonal and spatial variations in water quality in each sub-unit studied, which allowed the identification of a red contamination point within the ecosystem, coinciding with the geographical location of the city of San Miguel de Tucumán. The holistic vision achieved with spectroscopy detects the presence of organic molecules sliding through every system, without geographical or seasonal variations. It is a warning situation for the sustainability of the system and a potential threat that allows predicting their displacement in the aquatic environment (network effect); transforming a local contamination problem into a regional contamination problem. The evidence collected defines a ubiquitous behavior of the molecules, which means that they can be present in many places of the ecosystem, remain in the abiotic component, move to other geographical points or impact on different levels of the biotic component. In short, there is a danger of entry into urban areas, with water and also with food. The researches referred to Farm-ecovigilance that endorse as scientific background the objective of this Doctoral Thesis emphasize the concentrations, measured in micrograms, of IFA found in water in a natural ecosystem. This concept minimizes the threat posed by their mere presence, minimizes the effects they can produce. Moreover, their continuous input allows understanding temporal variations, even within 24 h. The threat of fulfilling a vicious cycle when reentering human populations is present, and they can be responsible for short, medium and long term effects on vulnerable populations, which poses a situation of uncertainty [Quesada, 2009]. In this study, hydrocarbon molecules were detected in water. The structure of its molecules ranges from the simplest represented by methane to those of greater complexity represented by polycyclic aromatic hydrocarbons. The organic molecules detected would be the subject of future pharmacovigilance studies to identify them by HPLC coupled to mass spectrometry. This methodology would allow the identification of circulating organic matter and with these drug spectra we should build a reference bank to identify analytes. This bank is fed with information obtained from drug utilization studies, which provide information on the most widely used drugs. The 1996 General Environmental Guide approved by the Secretariat of Natural and Human Resources of the Argentine Republic establishes that the environmental impact assessment (EIA) must include a monitoring plan and pharmacoecovigilance activities respond to this request. The pharmaco-ecovigilance monitoring plan defines an integrated work because it is nourished by information produced in the pharmaco-epidemiological stage and in the pre-clinical stage. The pre-clinical stage provides information on the behavior of the drug in the natural environment, for example, toxicity indexes (they serve as a reference to evaluate the concentrations detected in the environment under study). The information provided by pharmaco-epidemiological studies and pre-clinical studies can identify the drugs that represent the greatest risk to the natural eco-system. On this basis, regulate their use in the population and carry out controls. Liposoluble drugs, due to their chemical characteristics, represent a threat of deposition in the different hierarchical levels of the biota.

By bio-accumulation, they enter the food chain, with the danger of bio-magnification. Knowledge of the environmental toxicity of drugs, with

Pharmacological Profile and potential kinetic behavior of each drug based on its lipo- or hydrosolubility, allows designing pharmaco-ecovigilance actions and prevention measures during the epidemiological stage. Also, to promote rational use of the drug in question and to guide the search when these molecules are found in the environment. The construction of a Pharmacoecovigilance Monitoring Plan shows the value of systemic thinking in management. It allows articulating areas of study of pharmacological science, in a unit with interacting and interdependent parts. Farm-ecovigilance research in an aquatic ecosystem achieves new contributions related to the harmfulness of a drug. When it enters the natural ecosystem, it behaves as a pollutant, toxic to humans.

The threat of re-entry of molecules with water or food into the riverine human population is an inadvertent exposure that mobilizes Ecological Medicine. The response to environmental agents is variable, with age groups more susceptible and vulnerable than others. Industrialized countries attribute between 25 - 33% of diseases to environmental factors and the most vulnerable groups are children and pregnant women exposed on a daily basis. In addition, the fetus is exposed to other substances already stored in maternal tissues and chronic exposure is more worrying than acute exposure. However, the impact of IFAs present in the environment is poorly studied. The toxicity of drugs on the fetus has different consequences, depending on the time of exposure. Four main periods can be distinguished: the first 2 weeks, the period of organogenesis, the period of growth and differentiation, and the prepartum period. In addition to the teratogenic effects, there are reversible or permanent functional or biochemical or histological disorders, which are generally not accompanied by macroscopic morphological alterations. These functional alterations can be much more serious than anatomical malformations. For example, deafness or mental disorders are much more serious than a cleft lip. Emerging IFA pollutants, even at very low concentrations, can act as endocrine disruptors and alter the body's balance through endocrine dysfunction. Animal studies have demonstrated mechanisms that influence the hormonal system. These substances can totally or partially mimic natural hormones, e.g. estrogens, androgens, thyroid hormones. They modify intercellular communication and act as agonists or antagonists against a specific receptor. The impact of these pollutants has been verified by considering a) the dramatic effects seen in wild animals and their eco-systems b) the increase in the incidence of certain human diseases related to endocrine disorders c) the changes produced in experimental animals when tested with pollutants isolated from the environment surrounding the affected species. According to WHO, endocrine disruptors are chemical in nature, including persistent organic pollutants, pesticides, active ingredients in pharmaceuticals, additives, personal care products, cosmetics, etc. Inadvertent exposure to these molecules justifies continuous protective actions that should be part of health programs. In addition, chemical contaminants can produce epigenetic effects due to modification of gene expression, without changing the DNA code. The marks are produced in chromatin and can be transmitted to subsequent generations. The pharmacological groups whose residues are of greatest concern are antibiotics, antiparasitics, antifungals due to their greater use; also, antineoplastics and all those with high persistence in the environment. Public Health management requires green logistics, with the purpose of "*facing the challenge of reducing emissions*" and monitoring the environment, as a macro-strategy to be developed. It represents the set of initiatives aimed at analyzing and reducing the negative impact of pharmaceuticals on the environment [Petrovic et al. 2003]. Green logistics opens up healthcare spaces, technical-scientific departments, control, audit and teaching departments in the fields of drug use. It requires a new health professional profile that integrates research, teaching and auditing as postgraduate training for pharmacists, nurses, doctors and dentists. The responsibility of university educational institutions to include in their offerings, training programs for health professionals trained to perform in a new work scenario, increases in urban areas of higher population density, with a predominance of older adults, important consumers of medicines. A health management that responds to a green logistics, has hospitals, sources of urban pollution with a profile of the so-called green hospitals, which seek to continuously reduce their environmental impact and eliminate their contribution to the burden of disease. It recognizes the relationship between human health and the environment and demonstrates this through its management, strategy and operations. It connects local needs with environmental action and exercises primary prevention by actively participating in initiatives to promote community environmental health, health equity and a green economy. Educational activities aimed at promoting the rational use of medicines are part of a health management with green logistics, and represent a fundamental strategy to reduce emissions, the educational intervention must be carried out in the health care system, in the structure known as the medicine chain. These actions involve various actors: pharmaceutical industry, health professionals, user population. The general objective is to promote the development of eco-efficient processes to achieve therapeutically effective results at the lowest environmental cost, minimizing the environmental footprint of pharmacological origin. The new approaches in Public Health should control the pharmaceutical industry, forcing it to sustainable production with minimal generation of waste and polluting emissions [Agenda 2030 for Sustainable Development]. The pharmaceutical industry must provide information obtained in the preclinical stage and referred to the harmfulness of the drug on the natural eco-system. It should also assume responsibility for closing the life cycle of the active ingredient of the drug (from cradle to grave), applying reverse logistics, which involves planning, implementation and efficient control processes to ensure proper disposal. Pharmacoecovigilance shows that Public Health management needs to be developed in hospital and out-of-hospital settings, in order to educate and control. The lack of efficacy on non-biodegradable organic molecules presented by wastewater treatment plants requires the implementation of effective procedures for wastewater treatment. The elimination of seven carbadox antibiotics, trimethoprim and 5 classes of sulfonamides was studied with physicochemical treatments using polymers with aluminum sulfate ($Al_2 (SO)_{43}$ -$14H_2$ O) and ferric sulfate (Fe_2 (SO $)_{43}$ -$4H_2$ O). Huerta-Fontela et al. (2011) studied the removal of 35 pharmaceuticals and hormones using a coagulation/flocculation process followed by sand filtering. There are also studies that used other adsorbents, such as zeolites or carbon nanotubes, sugar cane bagasse, cocoa shells, among others [Prado 2010]; [Acero 2012]. Membrane technologies [Tambosi, 2010], nanofiltration (NF) and reverse osmosis (RO) [Kimura 2004] have also been used to remove emerging contaminants, which have been effective for some micropollutants resistant to conventional methods. Another process used for removal of emerging contaminants is ozonation [Gogate and Pandit 2004; Broséus et al. 2009; Rivas et al. 2012; Rosal et al. 2010], due to its high oxidation potential, or the use of hybrid technologies, such as membrane bioreactors (MBR). There are also examples of combined processes as disposal methods [Patiño et al. 2014]. There is a legal framework that mobilizes Public Health actions: the Precautionary Principle. It is a concept that supports the adoption of protective measures in the face of well-founded suspicions of a threat to the environment and that put public health at risk. For example, the presence of APIs in river water requires action to be taken even in a situation of scientific uncertainty and appropriate measures to prevent damage. This principle has established itself as a political and legal element in many countries, especially at the European and international levels. The principle represents a valuable tool in the configuration of a new paradigm for public policies required by present and future challenges. Pharmacoecovigilance monitoring contributes to achieving stable ecosystems and, by monitoring the state of an ecosystem, it defines prevention in human health, based on a culture of sustainable development [Delgado de Bravo 1996]. The detection of the presence of persistent organic molecules in watershed water represents the first step in farm-ecovigilance controls to identify active pharmaceutical ingredients.

Our results are pioneering and an important contribution to the care of Environmental Health with direct impact on Public Health.

7.4 Bibliography

Acero J., Benitez F.J., Real FJ., Teva F. (2012). Coupling of adsorption, coagulation, and ultrafiltration processes for the removal of emerging contaminants in a secondary effluent. Chemical Engineering Journal. 210, 1-8

2030 Agenda for Sustainable Development.

APHA, 1998. Standard Methods for Examination of Water and Wastewater. Clesceri L. S., Greenberg A. E. and Eaton A.D (Eds.). American Public Health Association - American Water Works Association - Water Pollution Control Federation, Maryland.

Barceló D. and López, M. J. Contamination and chemical quality of water: the problem of emerging pollutants. In: Scientific-Technical Panel for monitoring water policy. Instituto de Investigaciones Químicas y Ambientales-CSIC. 2007. Barcelona.

Barceló D., Petrovic M. (2007). Pharmaceuticals and personal care products (PPCPs) in the environment: Analytical and Bioanalytical Chemistry, 387, 1141- 1142.

Barron J., Ashton C., 2005. The Effect of Temperature on Conductivity Measurement. A Reagecon technical paper

Becerril J. (2009). Emerging Contaminants in Water. In: Revista Digital Universitaria 10 (8), 1-7.

Beltran, Luis. Turbidity, flocculation and sedimentation of water. 12 12 2011. http://procesosdeclarificaciondelagua.blogspot.com/ (last accessed 06 10 2018).

Broséus R., Vincent S., Aboulfadl K., Daneshva A., Sauvé S., Barbeau B., Prévost M. (2009). Ozone oxidation of pharmaceuticals, endocrine disruptors and pesticides during drinking water treatment. Water Res. 43, 4707-4717.

Cronon W. (1992). Nature's Metropolis: Chicago and the Great West. WW Norton and Company. New York-London

Dang H., Zhang X., Song L., Chang Y., Yang G. (2007). Molecular determination of oxytetracycline-resistant bacteria and their resistance genes from mariculture environments of China. Journal of applied microbiology. 103(6), 2580-2592.

Delgado de Bravo MT, (1996). Environment and Quality of Life. A response to the problems of the Latin American Metropolis. Buenos Aires. 6th Meeting of Latin American Geographers.

Delgado, S. Evaluation of potential technologies for the reduction of water pollution in the Canary Islands (tecnoagua). Project University of La Laguna, 2011

Gil M.J., Soto A.M., Usma J.I. and Gutiérrez O.D. (2012). Emerging contaminants in waters, effects and possible treatments. Cleaner production 7, 52-73.

Gogate, P. and Pandit, A. (2004). A review of imperative technologies for wastewater treatment I: oxidation technologies at ambient conditions. Advances in Environmental Research. 8, 501-551.

González-Pleiter, M., Cirés, S., Hurtado-Gallego, J., Leganés, F., Fernández-Piñas, F., Velázquez, D. 2019. Ecotoxicological assessment of antibiotics in freshwater using cyanobacteria. In: Mishra, A.K., Tiwari, D.N., Rai, A.N. (eds.), Cyanobacteria, pp. 399-417. Academic Press, India.

Grenni, P., Ancona, V., Caracciolo, A.B. 2018. Ecological effects of antibiotics on natural ecosystems: A review. Microchemical Journal 136:25-39.

Huerta Fontela M., Galceran MT., Ventura F. (2011). Occurrence and removal of pharmaceuticals and hormones through drinking water treatment. Water Res 45(3), 1432-42.

Kimura K, Toshima S, Amy G, Watanabe Y. (2004). Rejection of neutral endocrine disrupting compounds (EDCs) and pharmaceutical active compounds (PhACs) by RO membranes. J Membr Sci. 245(1), 71-8.

Kolpin D, Furlong ET, Meyer MT, Thurman EM, Zaugg SD, Barber LB, Buxton HT (2002). Pharmaceuticals, Hormones, and other Organic Wastewater 72 Contaminants in U.S. streams, 1999-2000: A national reconnaissance. Environ. Sci. Technol. 36, 1202-1211.

Kovalakova, P., Cizmas, L., McDonald, T.J., Marsalek, B., Feng, M., Sharma, V.K. 2020. Occurrence and toxicity of antibiotics in the aquatic environment: A review. Chemosphere 126351.

Larsson, D.J. 2014. Antibiotics in the environment. Upsala journal of medical sciences 119(2):108-112.

Lindström A., Buerge I., Poiger T., Anders Bergqvist P., Muller M., Buser H. (2002). Occurrence and environmental behavior of the bactericide triclosan and its methyl derivative in surface waters and in wastewater. In: Environmental science & technology 36 (1), 2322-2329.

Patiño Y., Díaz E., Ordóñez S. (2014). Emerging micropollutants in waters: types and treatment systems. Advances in Science and Engineering 5, 1-20.

Petrovic M; González S. and Barceló D. (2003). Analysis and removal of emerging contaminants in wastewater and drinking water. Trends in Analytical Chemistry 22, 685-696.

Pichett ST, Burch WR, Dalton SE, Foresman TW, Grove JM, Rowntree R, (1997). A conceptual framework for the study of human ecosystems in urban areas. Urban Ecosystems 1, 185-199.

Prados, G. Water treatment for the removal of Antibiotics, Nitroimidazoles by adsorption on activated carbon and advanced oxidation technologies. 2010. Thesis, Department of Inorganic Chemistry, University of Granada, Spain.

Quesada I, Jáuregui UJ, Wilhelm AM, Delmas H (2009). Water contamination with pharmaceuticals. Strategies to face the problem. Revista CENIC Biological Sciences 40, 173-179.

Rapport D.J., Costanza R., McMichael A.J. (1998). Assessing ecosystem health. Trends in ecology & evolution 13(10), 397-402.

Rapport D., Hildén M., Weppling K. (2000). Restoring the health of the earth's ecosystems: A new challenge for the earth sciences. Episodes, 23(1), 12-19.

Ratola N., Cincinelli A., Alves A., Katsoyiannis A., (2012). Occurrence of organic microcontaminants in the wastewater treatment process. A mini review. J. Hazard. Mater 239- 240, 1-18.

Rivas, F.J.; Beltrán, F.J. and Encinas, A. (2012). Removal of emergent contaminants: Integrations of ozone and photocatalysis. J. Environ. Manag. 100, 10-15.

Rivera-Utrilla J., Sánchez-Polo M., Ferro-García M.A., Prados-Joya G., Ocampo-Pérez R. (2013). Pharmaceuticals as emerging contaminants and their removal from water. A review. Chemosphere 93, 1268-1287.

Rosal R., Rodriguez A., Perdigón Melón JA., Petre A., García Calvo E., Gomez J., Aguera A., fernandez Alba AR. (2010). Ocurrence of emerging pollutants in urban wastewater and their removal through biological treatment followed by ozonation. Water Research 44 (2), 578-588.

Somsen G., Jagt T., Velthorst N., Brinkman U. (1996). Identification of hervicides in river water using on line trace inrichment combined whith column liquid chromatography-Fourier transform infrareel spectrometry. J. Chromatogr. A 756, 145-157.

Tambosi JL., de Sena RF., Favier M., Gebhardt W., Jose HJ., Schroder F., Muniz Moreira RF. (2010). Removal of pharmaceutical compounds in membrane bioreactors (MBR) applying submerged membranes. In: Desalination. 261, 148-156.

Valdés ME, Amé MV, Bistoni MDLA, Wunderlin DA (2014). Occurrence and bioaccumulation of pharmaceuticals in a fish species inhabiting the Suquía River basin (Córdoba, Argentina). Sci Total Environ. 472, 389-396.

Chapter 8

Conclusions

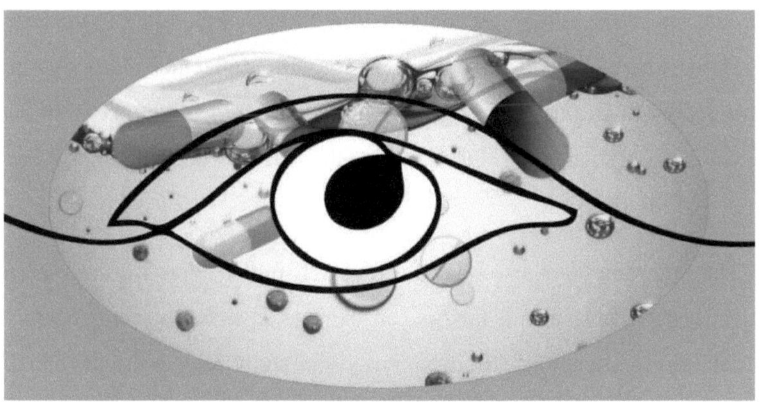

8.1 Conclusions
8.2 Contributions and Projections
8.3 Ecological glossary

8.1 CONCLUSIONS

- The decrease and loss of the biological self-purification capacity detected in the eco-system delimited in 100 km, belonging to the Salí Dulce watershed and the presence of organic molecules that move in it, represent an alert that forces to continue the study of this eco-system, with a transcendental function for the life of this region of the Argentine Republic.

- The microbiota is essential for the self-purification of the water ecosystem, but several factors can damage it, acting synergistically. The physical-chemical studies carried out show temporal and spatial variation in the state of the microbiota in the 100 km studied.
- The sub-ecosystem in direct contact with urban drainage is the most affected, as it has lost its biological self-purification capacity. In the other delimited ecosystems, biological self-purification is also compromised, which expresses a state of stress that affects sustainability.
- A local sanitary problem of chemical contamination, produced by the drains of a city, became a regional problem, with the danger of the appearance of local and networked adverse effects.
- The sensitivity of techniques such as Fourier transform infrared spectroscopy and atomic spectrometry allowed confirming the presence in the system under study of inorganic chemical compounds (Pb) and organic chemical compounds with potential harmfulness to the ecosystem, whose identification is in progress.
- In view of the limitations of the conventional methods used in urban wastewater treatment plants and water purification plants, in the face of the problem of pharmaco-pollution of the environment, other strategies such as the regulation of drugs that are harmful to the

environment, education to promote rational use and control with continuous monitoring programs become relevant.

- The systemic approach used to design and execute this research work was useful because it allowed the integration of different areas of science. From the environmental perspective, significant knowledge of the functioning of the subsystems studied was obtained, which will serve as a guide for other research related to the problem of pharmacological contamination and identification of biologically active molecules.
- Ecological Medicine is a preventive medicine, complementary to Clinical Medicine and Epidemiological Medicine.

8.2 CONTRIBUTIONS AND PROJECTIONS

The present work was a pioneer in the NOA region regarding the presence and behavior of the drug in a natural environment, thus extending the process of studying a drug.

The drug, transformed into a chemical residue of the drug, reaches the natural environment after being used by a population. This shows that the pharmaceutical product does not close its life cycle at the pharmaco-epidemiological stage.

The study process was developed in a space that transcends the limits of pharmacological science, where theoretical frameworks and methods of ecology were used, making this new space an inter-discipline: ***Pharmacoecology***. It is a holistic view, which managed to articulate the knowledge generated in previous stages of the study of a drug, with the knowledge in process, and to integrate pharmacology with other specialties, erasing disciplinary boundaries. The use of the eco-systemic approach to human health assumed by the General Theory of Systems surpassed the drug-medicine by also considering the environment where it is found and the effects that compromise health and life. The above mentioned bases the transversality of this new area of study with the Ecological Medicine, which takes care of the environment with a biocentric vision, protects life in all its expressions and is also the necessary complement of Clinical Medicine and Epidemiological Medicine. There is little information on the harmful effects of active pharmaceutical ingredients (API) on the natural environment. Neither is the effect of these pollutants on individuals and populations of fauna and flora, biological communities, species and on the ecosystems that host them known in depth. Some countries have biodiversity assessment studies, but they were not systematic, but rather the result of scattered and isolated efforts and initiatives with the fundamental purpose of detecting the APIs, identifying them and establishing their concentration. In general, the focus was on the pollutant, without considering that the damage to the biota breaks the balance of its ecosystem, an aspect highly valued by Ecological Medicine, since human health depends on the state of an ecosystem. The hydric eco-system, in which the research was initiated, is of great importance for the life of our NOA region. The interaction of two open systems was studied: the urban and the natural one in relation to the environmental impact of San Miguel de Tucumán's drains, which carry emerging pollutants, including IFA and agro-industrial wastes. The sub-ecosystem in contact with these drains is in a state of environmental distress, so it is necessary to work towards the transformation of San Miguel de Tucumán into a green city. The socio-scientific vision is crucial for the construction of this knowledge of pharmacological pollution of the environment. This socio-scientific vision places pharmacovigilance activities as a sanitary model of prevention, integrates it with pharmaco-epidemiological strategies, which promote the rational use of drugs and the regulation of the most dangerous APIs for the environment. It is important to emphasize that this is a group of unregulated pollutants. In relation to medicines, it is necessary to strengthen educational actions that emphasize the use of institutional drug formulations, to be used in sanitary spaces responsible for the greatest generation of chemical waste of pharmacological origin, such as hospitals, inducing the need for the so-called green hospitals. Sustainable practices and eco-efficient processes, during the production and use of the medicine, are the basis of environmental care. Eco-efficient processes should be implemented throughout the drug chain, with effective and environmentally cost-effective pharmacological interventions. The drug chain is a social system; its efficiency depends on political, economic and cultural influences, often at odds with the concepts of rational drug use, which transforms it into a danger to human, plant and animal health.

The results of this doctoral thesis work allowed, for the first time in the NOA region, to establish the right time and place to search for IFA. It also provided detection of organic molecules moving through the delimited ecosystem, whose uncertainty about their behavior encouraged future identification studies.

Our results show the need to apply the Precautionary Principle: "in case of threat to the environment or health and in a situation of scientific uncertainty, it requires that appropriate measures be taken to prevent harm". This scientific, pharmacoecological area has its own profile and deserves to be addressed in depth.

8.3 ECOLOGICAL GLOSSARY

Environment: set of external factors that act on an organism, population, community, influencing the survival, growth, development, reproduction of living beings, and the structure and dynamics of populations.

Biocenosis: (also called biotic community, biological community, ecological community or simply community) is the set of biological populations that coexist in space and time. These species occur in a defined space called biotope, which offers the environmental conditions necessary for their survival. It can be divided into phytocenosis (group of plant species), zoocenosis (group of animals) and microbiocenosis (group of microorganisms).

Biotope: (from the Greek βίος *bios*, "life" and τόπος *topos*, "place"), in ecology, is an area of uniform environmental conditions that provides living space for an assemblage of flora and fauna. Biotope is almost synonymous with the term habitat with the difference that habitat refers to species or populations while biotope refers to biological communities. A term that in the literal sense means living environment and applies to the physical, natural, limited space in which a biocenosis lives. The biocenosis and the biotope form an ecosystem.

Biodiversity is the variability among living organisms from all sources, including, inter alia, terrestrial and marine ecosystems and other aquatic systems, and the ecological complexes of which they are part; it includes diversity within species, between species, and of ecosystems.

Biocide: chemical substances used to control or destroy pests.

Biodegradable: applied to designate substances that can be degraded by the action of a biological agent.

Food chain: Sequential steps that organisms follow from producers to consumers, feeding at various trophic levels.

Pollutant load or mass load: measure representing the mass of pollutant per unit of time, which is discharged by a waste flow, expressed in Kg/d, T/day or Tons/year.

Water quality: is a term used to describe the chemical, physical and biological characteristics of water.

Environmental quality: represents the qualitative and/or quantitative characteristics inherent to the environment in general or particular environment, and its relation to the relative capacity of the environment to satisfy human and/or ecosystem needs. Environmental **quality** is measured by the health **of ecosystems** and their integrity. This environmental **quality** directly influences the health and way of life of society, although it is a concept that encompasses a large number of factors.

Biological cycle: The different stages through which an organism successively passes. It ranges from embryonic development and larval stages to offspring.

Community: biological conglomerate that includes all populations living in a given area.

Contamination: are the harmful modifications or alterations that environmental conditions undergo due to the presence of harmful elements or agents (physical, biological, chemical).

Contaminant(s): substance found in a medium to which it does not belong or whose presence is at levels that may cause (adverse) effects.

Ecosystem: any unit that includes all organisms in a given area interacting with the physical environment in such a way that a flow of energy leads to a clearly defined trophic structure, biotic diversity and material cycles. That is, an exchange of materials between living and non-living parts within the system is an ecosystem.

Network effect: network effect or network externality is used to describe situations in which the consumption of one population has negative consequences on others, thus regionalizing a local problem.

Eutrophication: Natural process in aquatic ecosystems, especially in lakes and rivers, characterized by an increase in the concentration of nutrients, with consequent changes in the composition of the living community.

Exposure: The contact of a population or individual with a chemical or physical agent. The magnitude of exposure is determined by measuring or estimating the amount (concentration) of the agent that is present on the contact surface (lungs, gut, skin, etc.) during a specified period.

Environmental impact: also known as anthropogenic impact or anthropogenic impact, is the alteration or modification caused by a human action on the environment. Since all human actions have an impact on the environment in some way, an environmental impact is differentiated from a simple effect by means of an assessment to determine whether the action carried out is capable of changing environmental quality.

Epidemiological profile: is the expression of the burden of disease (state of health) suffered by the population, and whose description requires the identification of the characteristics that define it. These characteristics include mortality, morbidity and quality of life.

Population: a group of organisms of the same species that reproduce freely among themselves and inhabit a given area.

Resilience: refers to the speed with which a community returns to its initial state after being disturbed by a disturbance and displaced from that state.

Biological System: A biological system is a complex network of biologically relevant entities. Biological organization spans several scales and is determined by different structures depending on the system.

Biological network: system based on subunits connected to each other within a whole, **e.g.**, trophic webs in an ecosystem, which allows the flow of energy.

Sustainability: that it can be sustained over time without depleting its resources or harming the environment.

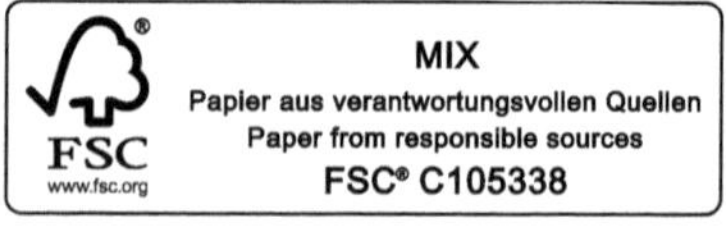

Printed by Books on Demand GmbH, Norderstedt / Germany